Personal but Not Private

PERSONAL BUT NOT PRIVATE

Queer Women, Sexuality, and Identity Modulation on Digital Platforms

Stefanie Duguay

OXFORD
UNIVERSITY PRESS

Oxford University Press is a department of the University of Oxford. It furthers
the University's objective of excellence in research, scholarship, and education
by publishing worldwide. Oxford is a registered trade mark of Oxford University
Press in the UK and certain other countries.

Published in the United States of America by Oxford University Press
198 Madison Avenue, New York, NY 10016, United States of America.

Library of Congress Control Number: 2022930691

ISBN 978-0-19-0-076191 (pbk)
ISBN 978-0-19-0-076184 (hbk)

DOI: 10.1093/oso/9780190076184.001.0001

9 8 7 6 5 4 3 2 1

Paperback printed by LSC Communications, United States of America
Hardback printed by Bridgeport National Bindery, Inc., United States of America

To mom, for your unrelenting love and support.

CONTENTS

ACKNOWLEDGMENTS

A quick Google search for the definition of *acknowledgment* returns two meanings: acceptance of the truth of something and expressing gratitude. Both meanings coalesce when I consider what it has taken to arrive on this page. The truth is that writing this book has only been possible thanks to the knowledge, effort, attention, care, resources, time, and countless contributions of many. This section is a brief attempt to express the gratitude that I hope to continue cultivating as a scholar, colleague, collaborator, friend, family member, and partner. My gratitude extends to an intention to also give back, and this book is one effort toward that.

Many thanks to those who I interviewed during this research and whose words and experiences inform this book. I appreciate your time and openness. Thank you more broadly to queer women who posted and continue to post on social media. As these pages attest, your self-representations are powerful in their world-making potential.

I would like to thank Oxford University Press, my editor Sarah Humphreville and editorial assistant Emma Hodgdon, the anonymous reviewers, copyeditors, and others who have logically, conceptually, and practically made this book possible. Some ideas, concepts, and findings in this book have appeared in previous publications, but all have been freshly revisited and examined here. Some interview excerpts in chapter 2 also appear in the following:

Ferris, L. & Duguay, S. Tinder's lesbian digital imaginary: Investigating (im)permeable boundaries of sexual identity on a popular dating app. *New Media & Society*, 22(3), pp. 489–506. Copyright © 2020 (Sage). doi:10.1177/1461444819864903

Duguay, S. "There's no one new around you": Queer women's experiences of scarcity in geospatial partner-seeking on Tinder. In C. J. Nash & A. Gorman-Murray (Eds.), *The Geographies of Digital*

Sexuality, pp. 93–114. 2019, Palgrave Macmillan. Reproduced with permission of Palgrave Macmillan.

Also, certain interview excerpts in chapters 3 and 4 appear in the following:

Duguay, S. "Running the numbers": Modes of microcelebrity labor in queer women's self-representation on Instagram and Vine. *Social Media + Society*, 5(4), pp. 1–11. Copyright © 2019 (Sage). DOI: 10.1177/2056305119894002

Duguay, S., Burgess, J., & Suzor, N. Queer women's experiences of patchwork platform governance on Tinder, Instagram, and Vine. *Convergence: The International Journal of Research into New Media Technologies*, 26(2), pp. 237–252. Copyright © 2020 (Sage). DOI: 10.1177/1354856518781530

Copyright © 2018 From "The more I look like Justin Bieber in the pictures, the better": Queer women's self-representation on Instagram by Stefanie Duguay. In Z. Papacharissi (Ed.), *A Networked Self: Platforms, Stories, Connections*, pp. 94–110. Routledge. Reproduced by permission of Taylor and Francis Group, LLC, a division of Informa plc.

Further, I have included references in the text to past publications upon which I expand in these chapters.

This research began during my PhD and owes a great deal to Jean Burgess for her careful guidance as well as to Ben Light and Elija Cassidy. I am thankful to the Digital Media Research Centre (DMRC) at the Queensland University of Technology (QUT) for enabling formal and informal discussions that contributed to these ideas. Thanks to my PhD cohort and the DMRC's researchers, lecturers, postdoctoral fellows, and visitors who provided great support as colleagues, collaborators, and friends, including (but surely not limited to) Pat Aufderheide, Axel Bruns, Xu Chen, Ella Chorazy, David Craig, Stuart Cunningham, Ehsan Dehghan, Michael Dezuanni, Frederik Dhaenens, Sara Ekberg, Ruari Elkington, Nikki Hall, Rachel Hews, Tim Highfield, Eddy Hurcombe, Katherine Kirkwood, Kelly Lewis, Ariadna Matamoros Fernández, Peta Mitchell, Silvia Montana Nino, Brenda Moon, Felix Muench, Kim Osman, Dan Padua, Emma Potter-Hay, Andrew Quodling, Aljosha Schapals, Fiona Suwana, Nicolas Suzor, Portia Vann, Jarrod Walczer, Patrick and Pia Wikström, Alice Witt, and Jing (Meg) Zeng. Portions of this research were made possible through QUT's financial support, including a Postgraduate Research Award, Higher Degree Research Tuition Sponsorship, Creative Industries Faculty Top-Up

Scholarship, and a Grant-in-Aid Travel Support Grant. The research analysis benefited greatly from the feedback of those on my confirmation and final seminar panels as well as the dissertation's examiners.

I was also fortunate to complete an internship at Microsoft Research's Social Media Collective (SMC) in the midst of this research. Thanks to Nancy Baym, Mary L. Gray, and Tarleton Gillespie for engaging discussions that furthered my understanding of science and technology studies, queer identity work, and platform governance. I am also appreciative of insightful discussions with the SMC members, other interns, postdoctoral fellows, and visitors, including Amelia Acker, Andrea Alarcón, Mike Ananny, danah boyd, Sarah Brayne, André Brock, Joan Donovan, Paul Dourish, Kevin Driscoll, Dan Greene, Caroline Jack, Shannon McGregor, Dylan Mulvin, Aaron Plasek, Lana Swartz, and Ming Yin.

This book's methods were informed by my participation in the Digital Methods Initiative's Summer Institute at University of Amsterdam. Thanks to Carolin Gerlitz, Anne Helmond, Bernhard Rieder, Richard Rogers, and Fernando Van Der Vlist for sharing your expertise. This training built upon the foundation I gained at QUT and at the Oxford Internet Institute, especially through Rebecca Eynon's guidance.

Concordia University has provided a rich academic environment for further working through the book's theoretical grounding. I would like to thank my colleagues in the Department of Communication Studies for their continued support. Thanks to Razan AlSalah, Mia Consalvo, Fenwick McKelvey, Liz Miller, and Alessandra Renzi for our discussions on topics of identity and digital media scholarship, as well as to Charles Acland and Monika Gagnon for your leadership and mentoring. Thanks to Krista Lynes for providing a welcoming space at the Feminist Media Studio for me to test ideas. Many thanks to the research assistants of the Digital Intimacy, Gender and Sexuality (DIGS) Lab and especially to Robert Hunt for his copyediting and formatting expertise. The final stages of this research have been facilitated by Concordia's Faculty Research Development Program Start-Up Fund and supported in part by funding from the Social Sciences and Humanities Research Council. I am appreciative of scholars in the wider Montreal and Canadian academic community, including members of the LabCMO and McGill University's Institute for Gender, Sexuality, and Feminist Studies, as well as global networks like the App Studies Initiative and the informal banter in the Hook-Up Apps Studies group.

While there are too many people to name as far as those who have impacted me over the course of writing this book, I wish to thank those in my extended academic family who have provided kindness, care, ideas, and support: Crystal Abidin, Kath Albury, Sophie Bishop, Rena Bivens,

Paul Byron, Christopher Dietzel, Amy Dobson, Elizabeth Dubois, Brooke Erin Duffy, Lindsay Ferris, Ysabel Gerrard, Amelia Johns, Amy Johnson, Alexandra Ketchum, Margaret MacDonald, Claudia Malacrida, Annette Markham, Cait McKinney, Mélanie Millette, Kate Miltner, Kristian Møller, Sharif Mowlabocus, David Myles, Emily van der Nagel, Susanna Paasonen, Thomas Poell, Brady Robards, Andrew Shield, Jenny Sundén, Lukasz Szulc, Katrin Tiidenberg, Son Vivienne, and more. Discussions with Katie Warfield contributed to this book and helped to make me the scholar and person I am today. I have much gratitude for the light and laughter she gave us in this world, which I know will endure through the many people she loved and inspired.

Friends across the world have been a great source of support. Thanks especially to Nick for the late-night snacks and enriching conversations. I am deeply grateful for the love of my family and my partner (and her family) throughout this whole process. Thanks, Bruce and Kristin, for your jokes that help to keep life in perspective and thank you Dennis—dad—for your ongoing support. Huge thanks to my mom, Bernice, who never doubted that I would write a book! Thank you, mom, for the hugs, phone calls, laughs, enthusiasm, listening, and love. Lastly, thanks to Jo, whose calmness and strength has always made this feel doable (and to our furbaby, Griffin, for his oversight and the occasional paw smash on the keyboard). Thanks, Jo, for letting me keep Tinder on my phone long after we met!

PROLOGUE

On July 22, 2012, I paced around my living room nervously. Thanks to Facebook's Timeline feature, I know this was the exact date.[1] I composed and recomposed a simple post, nearly deleting my draft attempts if it were not for Facebook's persistent question, "Do you want to leave without finishing?"

No. It had been several months since I started attending a local discussion group for bisexual people. Having found their information online, actually making my way to the group's small community-gathering space was an accomplishment, but it was also terrifying. I was not sure what others might share with me, let alone what I might learn about myself. I breathed, listened, and over the months eventually began to recognize resemblances between my experiences and those of other people in the room. I began to feel that identifying as bisexual helped me to make sense of my relationship to the world and other people in it. Increasingly, I wanted other people to know about my sexual identity—or, at least, to not be misread as heterosexual by default. But I didn't want it to be a big deal. I waited and then, eventually, a subtle yet purposeful reason to share about my sexual identity surfaced in my Facebook News Feed.

Someone from the discussion group shared a link to a research survey about bisexual people's mental health. I would like to think my then-latent academic inclinations contributed to my urge to share the link in service of advancing research. More realistically, my few bisexual Facebook friends would have already heard about the survey from our mutual contacts. Instead, sharing the link reflected how I wanted myself and my sexuality to be interpreted: a research-related post resonated with my unabashedly nerdy interests, and a study aiming to foster mental health and resilience among bisexual people seemed to fend off criticism in advance. Negative and biphobic responses to my coming out would be refuted as clearly part of the problem that surveys like this aim to address, right?

Despite this safeguard, I could feel my pulse accelerate as I stared at the post and contemplated my overlapping friend networks. As I would later see more vividly through network visualization activities in my graduate classes on digital research methods,[2] my connections cleaved into two distinct groupings: contacts from my hometown and those whom I encountered after leaving home. My hometown networks were dense. They included close and extended family, childhood friends, youth group contacts, and coworkers from my first part-time jobs. Partly due to the local culture of my prairie hometown in Western Canada, but also stemming from the messy process of trying out different identities and hobbies during my youth, this side of my network was heavily Christian and conservative in their values.

On the other side of this chasm were people I met when I moved into my first apartment in the relatively larger city of Ottawa. It is no secret that there is a long-standing trend of gay migration from rural areas to bigger cities, where nonheterosexual people find more people like themselves and benefit from more relaxed metropolitan attitudes toward sexuality (Sinfield, 1998). While this had not been my conscious motivation, since I never claimed a nonheterosexual identity in my hometown, living in a larger city with gay and lesbian venues, community centers, and Pride celebrations gave me the mental space to reflect on my sexuality. As such, I gravitated to people and organizations accepting of a diversity of sexual identities and eventually connected with some of my first openly lesbian, gay, bisexual, trans, and queer (LGBTQ) friends.[3] Simultaneously, I was also making connections with people at my first permanent, full-time job. Opinions at work ranged the full political spectrum, and although I became Facebook friends with some of my colleagues, I did not want to share anything too personal that could alienate me in such a new environment.

The cursor blinked in the status update box, already showing a preview of the survey web page. The words I typed are not seared in my memory, but they are enduringly available through Facebook's pristine archive: "Hey bisexuals (or people attracted to more than one gender and/or sex) in Ontario"—I believe this was the language used in the survey—"help out these researchers and help to improve mental health services for us." That was the key word: us. A word that could have been, and likely was, easily overlooked by many contacts as they skimmed their News Feed after dinner. And yet I felt it was straightforward, simple, and not in-your-face. I hit "Share" and called my mom.

I planned to use the Facebook post as a conversation starter with my mother. I understood that within hierarchies of disclosure, she should probably be the first to know since I was closer to her than anyone else in my life. However, I struggled to reach her. When I finally got through on her landline phone several hours later, more pressing family developments required attention, and I hung up without mentioning my post. Life proceeded as usual, and the post accrued a total of four "likes"—one from my male partner at the time and the rest from Ottawa contacts. I will never know who or how many people from my hometown saw this initial coming-out post over which I had agonized so painstakingly.

As I was about to be reminded, social media involve not only the posts we carefully curate and share but also others' responses, interactions, and occasional amplification of certain messages. Danah boyd (2014), a foundational scholar of social media, discovered this early in her discussions with youth, whose posts frequently signal developing aspects of identity. On social media platforms like Facebook or Twitter, identity is co-constructed as it is reflected through expressions building on norms and trends shared among people who form overlapping networks. However, boyd points out, posts can seem very strange when taken out of context.

The Monday following my anticlimactic survey post, my mom's coworker and good friend rushed into her office. It is important to note that my mom does not check Facebook regularly; she had not seen my post at all. What proceeded was a significant amplification and recontextualization of my post. They looked at it together as my mom's friend drew attention to the otherwise subtle wording indicating my sexual identity. The post was now framed in this conversation between them, involving questions of, "Did you know?"; "What do you think about that?"; and, inevitably, "Why didn't she tell you first?"

Spoiler alert: this experience fueled the curiosity with which I began to investigate how LGBTQ people come out and negotiate sexual identity on social media. Although my mom and I talked it out, and she has been an amazing support to me over the years, this instance gave me pause to reflect. Despite my friendship with my mom's coworker, she was not at the forefront of my mind as I formulated my post. I had not anticipated that Facebook's algorithms would surface the post in her feed or that she would pick up on my subtle wording and reframe it in an intense, in-person conversation. However, this was just the first of many instances that would draw my attention to the influential roles that platforms and their users play in shaping how people manage disclosures about sexual identity.

I say "disclosures" in the plural because coming out is not a single act, and social media platforms are often programmed to circulate what we share very widely. Following my survey post, I went on to share a portrait of my first "alternative lifestyle haircut," a defiantly asymmetrical bob that emulated queer fashion at the time. The cut embodied this term that

I had learned through the online magazine Autostraddle, which became responsible for most of my education about LGBTQ culture. Later, I posted politically charged articles about same-sex marriage debates and friends tagged me in photos after nights out at the local gay bar. I adjusted the privacy settings on these posts and maintained a separate Twitter account for professional contacts but mostly just allowed the rainbows to accumulate on my profile. I experienced firsthand how this digital reflection of my sexual identity could do the work of coming out for me: friends across oceans noticed when I posted selfies with a woman and wrote to confirm their hunches that I had a girlfriend. When I returned to my hometown and had lunch with a former colleague, she remarked bluntly, "So, you're a lesbian now."

I want to be clear though, the stakes for my coming out have been pretty low. I was already financially independent and employed, my parents have been accepting, and I traverse life with the privilege society affords to white, cisgender people. A few Facebook contacts from back home have dropped off over the years, but this could have been due to our lack of interaction as much as any offense they may have taken. I am well aware that there are people who must be much more covert about their disclosures of sexual identity due to threats of being disowned by their families, workplace discrimination, homophobic attacks, and even death sentences. As this book examines the complications that social media invoke for managing information about sexual identity, it is certainly important to reflect on how our current technological arrangements can put these individuals in grave danger. These are the instances when confusing privacy settings or cross-platform data sharing can be life shattering.

However, this book is about people who post about their sexual identity on social media in ways that appear to be fairly overt. Similar to my accumulation of rainbows, I approached many of my interview participants specifically because their social media clearly reflected LGBTQ identities. Their posts were not secret, they were not private, but a lot of the time they were personal in the information about sexual identity that they conveyed. I argue that these kinds of everyday, personal posts matter because of the capacity they hold for enabling queer women to connect with others; to form publics for social and economic participation; and to counter sexual and gender stereotypes, biases, and discrimination. In order to put themselves out there like this, these women required the ability to influence multiple aspects of how they presented their sexual identity on social media. They also needed a degree of control over which audiences would receive and respond to these presentations. As we will see, without these capabilities, the women I spoke with felt that their social media activity became ineffective and subject to misinterpretation and harassment.

Further to the opportunities for self-development and social connection that are lost when LGBTQ individuals cannot be visible on social media, every single person has a right to determine how they present themselves and how far their personal information travels. Since I started teaching, I have set my Instagram account to "private." Not to hide anything in particular but mostly so my students remain separated from my social snapshots and stylized landscapes. However, my partner tagged me in a selfie one day, and I remember asking from the living room, "Does that mean that everyone can see my name tagged, since your account is public?" Even as a social media scholar, I cannot keep up with all the features and functions that stymie our agency over self-representation. As many scholars and opinion leaders have begun to argue for greater user autonomy over data, my aim with this book is for us to remember that for a lot of people, their data include personal expressions: identity statements, first kisses, relationship commitments, and declarations of solidarity with marginalized or targeted groups. For LGBTQ people, the personal is something that society has historically constructed as private, carrying consequences for people's freedom and well-being if it becomes public. This book examines ways that social media both obfuscate and enable personal expressions that hold powerful ramifications for individuals' lives as well as public change.

CHAPTER 1

Digital Mediations of Sexual Identity and Personal Disclosure

Phyllis gave a loud sigh and plunked her iced tea on the table between us. We were early into the interview, and I had only asked standard demographic questions so far. The latest was, "How would you describe your sexual identity?" I watched the condensation roll down the sides of her beverage—evidence of another sweltering day in Queensland, Australia—and waited as she responded reluctantly, "I'm probably a lesbian—that seems best." She settled on this descriptor to satisfy my question but quickly discounted it, "I'm pretty boring; that's all I am."

I nodded noncommittally, not wanting to invalidate her sentiment. As a queer-identified woman dedicated to researching LGBTQ people's use of social media, clearly I did not find lesbians boring, but I kept this to myself. I worried that the rest of the interview might also be interspersed with sighs, but Phyllis became more animated as soon as I asked her to open the dating app Tinder on her phone. Proud of the witty one-liner self-description she had fit into her profile, she read it aloud, "I excel at dank memes, lesbianing and getting my law assessments done six weeks in advance." She turned the screen toward me and exclaimed, "That's me." The description was followed by three emoji: a peace sign, a rainbow, and two women holding hands (✌️ 🌈 👭).

There was a lot packed into this short declaration. Phyllis had managed to demonstrate her humor, with the reference to "dank memes" as a self-effacing passion for overdone jokes, and to humblebrag about the diligence with which she was completing a challenging university degree. Couched within this description was a reference to the sexual identity she

Personal but Not Private. Stefanie Duguay, Oxford University Press. © Oxford University Press 2022.
DOI: 10.1093/oso/9780190076184.003.0001

had lamented earlier as inconsequential. When I asked why she had decided to include these details, her response focused on this identifier, "The 'lesbianing' thing—it's from *Orange Is the New Black* and, just in case they didn't get that I was gay from the rainbows, they're like, 'No, she's definitely gay. She's a lesbian. She said she's good at lesbianing.'"

Netflix's comedy-drama prison show *Orange Is the New Black* (2013–19) was hitting peak popularity when I conducted these interviews in 2016. The lead character, Piper, had relationships with both men and women, and although the show shied away from giving her a bisexual label (Ferguson, 2016), other characters openly identified as lesbian. In episode 9 of the first season, a redneck-stereotyped character, nicknamed Pennsatucky, tells a corrections officer that Piper and her ex-girlfriend are engaging in "lesbian activity," in fact, "they lesbianing together." Fans quickly spread this short, catchy phrase online (see figure 1.1), though it faded in popularity as the show continued. Phyllis's self-description of her sexual identity was itself a dank meme.

Personal but Not Private is about these instances on social media, in which putting one's sexual identity out there for others to see becomes

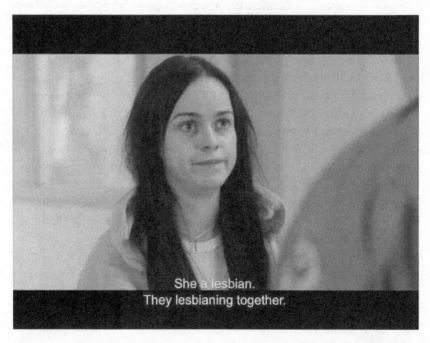

Figure 1.1 *Orange Is the New Black* character Tiffany "Pennsatucky" Doggett telling Officer Healy about Piper's sexual dancing with ex-girlfriend Alex Vause. Source: u/orionlady, Lesbianing. Posted on August 20, 2013. https://www.reddit.com/r/actuallesbians/comments/1ks5yh/lesbianing/.

important. In the context of our interview, it did not matter to Phyllis whether I wrote down that she identified as lesbian or anything else—I was just an interviewer. She had mostly signed up for the interview because her friend told her it would be fun to chat about Tinder. But I would later learn that Phyllis declaring herself a lesbian on Tinder was a significant choice within the app's framing and in light of its users. This declaration served to attract the types of matches she considered date-worthy, while Tinder's settings and swipe features were not sufficient for achieving this alone.

The analyses presented throughout this book demonstrate that queer women's representations of sexual identity become important because they serve particular purposes on different social media platforms, whether these purposes comprise partner seeking, the accrual of capital, or rallying others around a collective statement. Sexual identity may not be something that all people feel the need to mention in casual, everyday interactions. For some people like Phyllis, who even in her early twenties had been out to her acquaintances for years and who moves with ease across many social situations due to elements of privilege like white skin and upper-middle-class status, sexual identity is inconsequential in many contexts. For others, conditions of homophobia or intersectional discrimination may limit their ability to express their sexual identity at all. However, one only needs to run a few searches on popular platforms to see a volume of content by individuals showcasing lesbian, gay, bisexual, transgender, queer (LGBTQ),[1] and other diverse gender and sexual identities. I argue that many of these self-representations are intentional, instrumental, curated, and ultimately modulated in conjunction with platform mechanisms in attempts to invoke particular outcomes.

Self-representation has the potential to be extremely powerful. I use the term *self-representation* to describe how ordinary—that is, everyday—people create mediated texts with the potential for subsequent engagement (Thumim, 2012). While self-*presentation* can be thought of as more generally as something that we may do passively or in response to others, self-*representation* holds greater agency, often involving premeditated and intentional ways of representing oneself, and digital technologies can facilitate this. Individuals create mediated texts in the form of statements, photos, videos, and other kinds of posts, which others can view, circulate, and respond to as they take advantage of digital tools enabling collective creativity (Bruns, 2008; Jenkins, 2006). The queer women's self-representations you will encounter throughout this book include Tinder profiles similar to Phyllis's in their adornment with LGBTQ-related emoji, glamorous Instagram photos tagged with #girlswholikegirls, and long-lost Vine skits calling out homophobia. Through a combination of long-standing references to sexual identity, such as the rainbow flag, and forms of digital culture like hashtags, individuals choose how to include this personal and often intimate detail about themselves in their social media.

Of course, social media platforms' complex political, economic, sociocultural, and technological arrangements have a profound effect on their users' self-representations. These factors shape how content is produced and presented to others while also scaffolding the environments where interactions take place among users (Bucher, 2018; Gillespie, 2018; van Dijck, 2013). Platformed self-representations are not only the product of an individual's self-expression but also intrinsically tied to the digital formats, markets, and policies through which they are deployed. Self-representations of sexual identity combine with platform arrangements in particular ways, rubbing up against censorship policies or surfacing in the newsfeeds of forgotten acquaintances.

As the title suggests, this book is about how all of this comes together when something personal—specifically, sexual identity—is shared on social media in a way that is not private. For reasons I will explain, this book focuses on queer women: people whose gender is female and who are attracted to others who are also female. This definition understands gender as mutually constructed among individuals and society while acknowledging its range and fluidity, meaning that included in these pages are transgender, cisgender, gender nonconforming, feminine, and masculine women. I describe these women as queer due to their tension with heteronormativity and other normative systems of oppression that intersect with sexual identity (Warner, 1999). However, my findings are pertinent for everyone because social media encourage sharing—this is the default platform activity and a Silicon Valley mantra.

Scholars Zizi Papacharissi and Paige Gibson (2011) point out that we trade our privacy and personal information on social media in exchange for sociability. Both my previous research and several other studies have focused on how LGBTQ people who may not want to share widely information about their sexual identity develop strategies for keeping certain posts from the prying eyes of homophobic colleagues or family members (Duguay, 2016a; Hanckel et al., 2019). However, as I have looked closely at queer women's self-representations—examining their content, talking with them about their decision-making, and deeply investigating the platforms they use—it has become apparent that there is no easy compilation of digital literacy resources for managing personal sharing on social media. There is no heuristic, standard set of strategies or hack for your privacy settings. Instead, for people who manage a personal piece of information that can be both powerful and potentially stigmatizing if shared, there are multiple and ongoing approaches taken by the user, along with several platform affordances that come into play.

There are also many instances when platforms get in the way of these approaches, leading to self-representations being circulated more widely than intended or, conversely, rendered invisible. Notably, this book does not focus on maintaining sexual identity as private but on the important daily efforts that go into sharing personal information through social media to invoke meaningful outcomes. The book's framework of *identity modulation* provides a way to understand individual and platform roles in the management of personal information on social media.

IDENTITY MODULATION

"Modulate your voice!" my mother used to tell my brother and me when we were being rambunctious. This guidance was not merely a request for us to be quieter; otherwise she might have said, "Pipe down!" Instead, it was an invitation for us to consider the appropriate level of expression given our activity, the environment, and the people surrounding us. Whether in the backyard, at school, or at the dinner table, modulating my voice meant something different, and I adjusted accordingly. My resulting verbal expression was then a product of both my own agency and the shaping role of the social and material context.

Digital media scholar John Cheney-Lippold (2017) introduces the concept of modulation into the context of digital media technologies. He notes that the term holds a central idea of "dynamism and variance according to stability" (p. 101). Modulation reflects the capacity to adjust and change in relation to other factors that remain the same, such as my shift from an "outside voice" to a softer, more articulate utterance around the family dinner table.[2] Cheney-Lippold fleshes out this concept through philosopher Gilles Deleuze's (1992) description of modulation as the way that contemporary *societies of control* function. According to Deleuze, control mechanisms constantly modulate influential factors in people's lives, from exchange rates to salaries. Focusing on computational algorithms as a control mechanism, Cheney-Lippold asserts that as our identities have become datafied through the use of digital technologies, control is exerted upon us when the algorithms interpreting and defining our identities change— or modulate—in frequent and unknown ways. In his analysis, algorithms modulate identity categories built from large-scale data aggregation. This modulation then affects how we are targeted as consumers, are treated as citizens, and see ourselves while algorithms serve up responsive content through our platforms and devices.

Data and algorithms are certainly relevant to the experiences and arrangements of digital technologies discussed in this book. But I want to pick up on Cheney-Lippold's emphasis on modulation as dynamic, variant, and ever-changing, drawing on it to consider how both users and platforms can be forces of modulation. My research leads me to consider more widely how individuals, situated within particular histories and cultures of sexuality and digital media, interface not only with algorithms but also with multiple aspects of platforms' technological features, economic interests, and governance measures. Therefore, I build on science and technology scholarship that takes seriously the mutual shaping of users and technology to examine such modulation processes (MacKenzie & Wajcman, 1999; Sismondo, 2010).

To do so, I find it useful to return to the idea of sound modulation, which—after all—is what underlies the prompt to "modulate your voice!" The processing of sound waves provides an appropriate metaphor to guide us through what happens when individuals signal personal information on platforms. Modulation processes on a radio channel occur when an *input wave* is imposed on a *carrier wave* to encode it with information, such as speech or music (Tait Communications, 2019). The resulting combined sound wave is changed by the modulation process: it may have a different frequency—affecting the pitch—or an altered amplitude, making the sound louder or quieter. I sometimes liken identity modulation to adjusting the volume switch on one's self-representation. The individual presses the buttons, whereas the platform defines the boundaries of loudness or quietness. While I return to this connection with volume in chapter 3, the following section makes clear that identity modulation has multiple dynamics, so it is necessary to think about it beyond binary qualities such as loud or quiet.

Sound modulation is an entanglement between the sound and multiple actors involved in its processing. Cultural studies scholar Jonathan Sterne and music historian Tara Rodgers (2011) define signal processing as what "happens in the middle of media" (p. 35). The signal processing of sound waves takes place among musicians, playback technology, and listeners to the extent that when it "modulates recorded sound or music . . . the effects tend to be heard as inseparable from the sound and music itself" (p. 35). These scholars maintain that this inseparability makes signal processing, as the modulation of sound, difficult to critique and analyze.

Self-representation of sexual identity on social media has a similarly seamless quality. Sexual identity can be understood as a specific signal or input wave, which is communicated by, with, and through a platform—as a metaphorical carrier wave—in ways that modulate this information. While the individual has agency in crafting a self-representation and anticipating how the platform may shape it, platforms complicate individuals' approaches. This mutual shaping between the user and the platform is not usually discernible by the time a self-representation reaches one's social media audiences, who interpret the information within not just the platform's context but also the broader sociocultural meanings relating to sexuality.

Identity modulation pertains to the ongoing processes that shape the self-representation of an individual's personal information—sexual identity, in this case—in relation to social media audiences. It involves individual decision-making, in which judgment calls are made when pairing a potentially sensitive or stigmatized piece of personal information with other identifying information, such as one's legal name or visual likeness. However, identity modulation is also contingent on social media's features, functions, policies, and norms that make certain modes of action available (or more likely) over others. To understand how identity modulation is pivotal in arrangements among people and technology, it is necessary to consider, first, the sociocultural meaning of sexual identity as a specific kind of personal information and, second, the implications of disclosing this information through platforms and apps.

Sexual Identity as Personal, Not (Necessarily) Private

I understood sociologist Erving Goffman's (1963) definition of stigma long before ever reading his words. Growing up in the 1990s, I watched reruns of the iconic Canadian teenage drama *Degrassi Junior High* (1987–91) after school every day. The show covered an array of issues—from drugs to teen pregnancy—with a cast that was much more diverse than other television shows of the time. One episode, aptly named "Rumor Has It," remains etched in my memory. The main plotline goes like this: a teacher, Ms. Avery, is rumored to be a lesbian, and this worries Caitlin, a female student who keeps having dreams that vaguely indicate some attraction between her and Ms. Avery. Caitlin's friends eventually pick up on her worry and accuse her of also being a lesbian. This accusation leads her to snap at Ms. Avery, who then has a heart-to-heart with Caitlin in which Ms. Avery establishes she is not a lesbian after all. The episode's key challenge to the rumor is a question, echoed by one student throughout and by Ms. Avery at the end: "What difference would it make?" Through my preteen eyes, the answer was: a life-altering difference. Despite the show's attempt to address homophobia, the episode depicts suspected lesbian characters being teased, treated with disgust, and othered. It reinforces Goffman's (1963) definition of stigma as that which forges difference between people based on a discrepancy between assumptions about individuals and their actual qualities. The students assume everyone is, or should be, heterosexual, and so the prospect of Caitlin or Ms. Avery being different subjects them to stigma, enacted through words and actions that shame them.

Throughout the episode, the students find evidence for Ms. Avery's lesbianism, such as glimpses of her holding hands with friends and the fact that she lives with another woman. These scenes illustrate how "deviant" practices are understood to communicate something about identity. Philosopher Michel Foucault (1978/1990) traced a similar trajectory through religious, psychiatric, and medical institutions, uncovering how they incited people to connect sexual practices to labels or diagnoses. Through these institutions and the imperative they created for self-identifying with such labels, sexual identity became sticky, something that sticks to a person—it became personal. One of the episode's terrifying dream sequences illustrates this process of practices becoming associated with identity labels when Ms. Avery gives Caitlin a side hug and the other students chant: "Lesbian! Lesbian! Lesbian!"

Judgments of discrepancy and deviance rest on assumptions stemming from dominant cultural practices, perceptions, and values. Political scientist Cathy Cohen (2005) defines heteronormativity as the default assumption of heterosexuality, which also comes with gender roles and scripts. Connecting the dots between sex and gender, philosopher Judith Butler's (1990) "heterosexual matrix" highlights the widespread assumption that bodies have "a stable sex expressed through a stable gender . . . that is oppositionally and hierarchically defined through the compulsory practice of heterosexuality" (p. 208). This matrix dovetails with more recent understandings of cisnormativity as the assumption that an individual's biological sex characteristics at birth will match with associated traditional gender performances throughout one's life (Worthen, 2016). In the 1980s and early 1990s, Ms. Avery's single status and exuberant displays of encouragement to both female and male students ran counter to normative sexual and gender scripts.

Enough with my haunted memories; you may be thinking, aren't we past all this? After all, *Degrassi* has been remade multiple times with an increasing roster of LGBTQ characters. Indeed, in the subsequent decades since this episode's airing, there have been fairly successful political movements aiming for increased acceptance of homosexuality by downplaying difference (Warner, 1999). A reduction in difference pacifies stigma but is also limited in challenging the norms that instantiated difference in the first place. In the early 2000s, American studies scholar Lisa Duggan (2002) identified that greater tolerance of homosexuality was owed, in large part, to the emergence of a "new homonormativity" comprised of "a politics that does not contest dominant heteronormative assumptions and institutions but upholds and sustains them while promising the possibility of a demobilized gay constituency and a privatized, depoliticized gay culture anchored in domesticity and consumption" (p. 179). Years of "equal rights" campaigns have fought for LGBTQ people's integration into society as *normal* people. However, claims of normality must be demonstrated through adherence to dominant norms, such as marriage, monogamy, and domesticity (Warner, 1999). Homonormativity is no longer new. It has ushered in much greater LGBTQ representation in forms that no longer raise eyebrows thanks to an overarching emphasis on sameness. While Ms. Avery's question of whether homosexuality makes a difference seemed cutting-edge in the 1980s, this tired message replays across seasons of *Queer Eye* (2018–) in ways that affirm the importance of affluence and normative attractiveness in bids for acceptance.

Despite this trend toward downplaying difference, coming out—as a ritual of disclosing sexual identity—has not gone away. Institutions and social roles still call on individuals to claim a particular sexual identity, which allows for them to be categorized and rationalized into societal structures (Foucault, 1978/1990). As Goffman (1968) observed, people are expected to disclose their stigma in order to realign others' assumptions and avoid being discredited as lying or hiding what makes them different. But aside from seeming well adjusted or honest, coming out is also a step toward blending in. Within a neoliberal context that prizes individual rights and freedoms (Richardson, 2005), coming out enables some individuals to adopt normative identity scripts and forms of consumption that allow them to move through life much like anyone else. Nonheterosexuality is thus seen as an individual struggle that can be addressed through coming out, which allows LGBTQ people to transition into self-acceptance and recognition as consumer citizens.

Some scholars and media pundits posit that coming out and LGBTQ visibility may now be trivial matters. They assert that we have entered a "post-gay era," which allows an individual to dissociate from homosexual stereotypes and "define oneself by more than sexuality" (Ghaziani, 2014, p. 102). However, those who are most able to sidestep explicitly coming out quite often possess other qualities in alignment with dominant ideologies (such as patriarchy and white supremacy) and normative standards of ability and socioeconomic status (McNaron, 2007; Nash, 2013). That is to say, men who are white, able-bodied, and of high socioeconomic status have a much easier time than women, people of color, people with disabilities, and those with lower incomes in coming across as *normal*, even if they are gay. And as the term *post-gay* implies, sexual identities that have seen less integration into popular culture and less commercialization than (cisgender male) gay identities remain steeped in difference, which fuels stigma and necessitates coming out.

But coming out carries both transformative potential and risk. It could bring about changes in attitudes, institutions, and societal structures as it challenges heteronormativity. This capacity to facilitate change is especially potent when carried out collectively, such as through coalitional movements that attach gay or queer liberation to intersecting fights for freedom from racial and class discrimination (Cohen, 2005). This sort of confrontational coming out, however, carries the risk of punishment and backlash, from social isolation to discrimination. It also tends to involve grand gestures, occurring momentously when people choose to become involved in political moments.

Much more commonly, people come out in everyday moments, such as when I call to clarify my spouse's gender on shared bills. These moments can also be transformative, as acts of "everyday activism" (Vivienne, 2016a) that disrupt assumptions a little at a time, and they remain risky for the challenge they pose to the status quo. Refusing to erase difference means putting one's seamless participation in institutions of labor, the family, and consumption—the trappings of life within neoliberal citizenship—in peril. With these risks in mind, many LGBTQ people engage in what sociologist Jason Orne (2011) calls "strategic outness": a context-specific approach to determining whether or not to disclose one's sexual identity. As we will see, coming out happens through small and large gestures across platforms. While my *Degrassi* memories are rife with sweaty nightmare scenes of having to conceal sexual identity, a very different landscape of LGBTQ representation abounds across social media.

Digital Disclosure

To understand the role of social media platforms and apps in the disclosure of highly personal information, it is useful to return to Goffman's ideas, as many media scholars have done (Blackwell et al., 2015; Hogan, 2010; Lim et al., 2012; Papacharissi, 2009; Vitak, 2012). Goffman (1959) applied a dramaturgical model to social interactions, viewing individuals as actors in performances taking place across the different stages, or contexts, of our lives. He differentiated between front-stage performances—those tailored to particular audiences—and less curated expressions in backstage regions away from these audiences, which allow for performances to be relaxed, rehearsed, or even contravened. People experiencing stigma may be "living a life that can be collapsed at any moment" (Goffman, 1963, p. 109) should their stigmatized quality be revealed in front-stage regions. Communication scholar Joshua Meyrowitz (1985) identifies that electronic media alter these regions by dislodging social exchanges from their embeddedness in physical space. This gives rise to new social situations without such clean-cut boundaries for interaction, sometimes merging audiences or giving front-stage audiences a sneak peek at the backstage, such as when TV reporters conduct home interviews with politicians or celebrities.

Social media's affordances have the potential to disrupt these regions even further. One of the first scholars to examine teenagers' behavior on MySpace and later Facebook, danah boyd (2014) extends Meyrowitz's ideas to understand how social media present new opportunities and challenges for social interaction. She describes how social media facilitate "networked publics" that are "simultaneously (1) the space constructed through networked technologies and (2) the imagined community that emerges as a result of the intersection of people, technology, and practice" (p. 8). While I will reflect further on how identity modulation can give rise to networked publics in chapter 4, I wish to underscore boyd's observation that networked publics often bring together disparate audiences. She identifies social media as affording increased persistence, visibility, spreadability, and searchability to the content with which such audiences circulate and interact (though these affordances vary depending on the platform). As such, there is a much higher likelihood that front- and backstage regions will merge compared to earlier media formats. Boyd refers to this as "context collapse," which "occurs when people are forced to grapple simultaneously with otherwise unrelated social contexts that are rooted in different norms and seemingly demand different social responses" (p. 31). While stigmatized individuals are often already conscious of the potential for contexts to collapse, social media generate new situations with a high propensity for this to occur.

Fortunately, people can adapt their approaches to personal disclosure to deal with the possibility of context collapse. Since the audience for a social media post may be unknowable, especially on publicly searchable platforms like Twitter, individuals tend to tailor their expressions to an "imagined audience" (Marwick & boyd, 2011). Researcher Eden Litt (2012) describes the imagined audience as the "mental conceptualization" of others with whom one is interacting. She notes that this concept builds on Benedict Anderson's (1983) pivotal definition of "imagined communities" being comprised of those who may not be known in person but with whom one assumes a shared commonality or connection, such as among citizens of the same nation. Therefore, social media users employ their skills and motivations to craft posts that resonate most with the audiences they imagine as their ideal recipients. Teenagers often post lyrics or other encoded texts that only mean something to particular audiences (Marwick & boyd, 2014). On YouTube, many creators adjust access to their videos in relation to the level of personal detail included in them (Lange, 2007). These examples reflect strategies for targeting audiences and adjusting the level of information disclosed.

When people tailor their self-representations, they tend to view a platform as a specific social context, reconstructing the boundaries of this particular stage. Studies of teenagers' disclosures on social media reveal that they deploy personal information in alignment with a platform's social norms—that is, they anticipate that others will view and interpret their posts within the platform's context (Livingstone, 2008; Marwick & boyd, 2014). This practice highlights a definition of privacy as "having control over who knows what about you" (Livingstone, 2008, p. 404). This definition resonates with contemporary understandings of privacy as functioning in relation to norms that govern personal information flows in social contexts (Nissenbaum, 2009). Information scientist Helen Nissenbaum (2009) asserts that new technologies often violate such "contextual integrity" as they disrupt these information norms, often distributing information beyond what people perceive to be the context for their sharing. Seeming eerily predictive of today's social media, Meyrowitz (1985) similarly identified the importance of information flows, noting: "The dividing line between backstage and onstage is informational, not necessarily physical" (p. 39). Privacy, then, becomes a matter of managing what other people know about you and maintaining the context for this information, ensuring that it reaches intended audiences and not others.

These approaches to maintaining privacy, in the sense of *who* knows *what*, are common throughout this book. However, my main concern is not with the management of privacy but with what is disclosed. I focus on how such information is deployed, shaped by the platform, and received by others. I want to note, though, that personal disclosures on social media are not often public, if we think about publicness as the flip side of a contextual definition of privacy. If public information is intended for viewing across multiple contexts, audiences, and interpretative norms, then the personal information shared in specific platform contexts constitutes something different.[3] The disclosures of sexual identity throughout this book are not private, in the sense of being locked down or suppressed, but nor are they public in this broader sense. They are personal: shared through particular symbols, resonating with specific audiences, and intended to evoke certain outcomes when communicated in ways that include an element of control over their delivery.[4]

Similar to how the multiple elements of signal processing are indiscernible when a fully mastered sound is produced, self-representations of identity on social media often appear as personal expressions without immediately noticeable platform influences. However, in relation to networked publics, privacy also becomes networked, since platforms' features and functions are always changing in tandem with evolving user norms and fluctuating audiences (Marwick and boyd, 2014). Further, new media scholar José van Dijck (2013) argues that platforms are microsystems of constitutive elements that shape sociality. These elements include users, technology, and content as platforms' "techno-cultural constructs" (p. 28), and they feature prominently in those studies of networked publics and context collapse mentioned earlier. But van Dijck also identifies elements that comprise platforms' "socioeconomic structures" (p. 28), including their ownership, governance, and business models. Recognizing these multiple elements of platform influence enables a nuanced examination that moves beyond the initial seamlessness of a Tinder profile, Instagram photo, or Vine video to identify how individuals and platforms together form these reflections of identity.

Identity modulation is a process by which people, together with platforms, negotiate the gray area between being private and public with personal information. On the user's side, identity modulation involves disclosure through approaches that tailor content to imagined audiences within a platform's context. Beyond approaches to preserving privacy, identity modulation is very much about putting personal information *out there*. Platforms shape these disclosures through much more than their features and functionality, as their economic imperatives and governing decisions also affect individuals' self-representations. As something that is not entirely considered public or private, sexual identity is an apt quality through which to examine identity modulation. There is an imperative to come out in order to participate fully in social and economic life, and yet nonheterosexuality is still often relegated to private spaces to downplay its difference from heterosexuality. As a digitally mediated process through which indicators of personal, potentially stigmatized identifiers are deployed and treated on platforms, identity modulation is not necessarily limited to displays of sexual identity. However, LGBTQ people's legacy of managing the information they convey is useful for understanding how digital technologies shape processes of disclosure.

DYNAMICS OF IDENTITY MODULATION

In some senses, identity modulation is not new. Individuals have been making decisions about how and to whom they present their personal information for a very long time. Similarly, digital technologies have shaped these processes in all sorts of ways over recent decades. Returning to the metaphor of sound, recall that modulation can affect a sound wave's frequency or amplitude. In terms of personal disclosure, identity modulation alters certain dynamics relating to the communication of personal information. These dynamics include (a) *personal identifiability*, as the other identifying information conveyed alongside the personal disclosure; (b) the *reach* of a personal disclosure across audiences and platforms; and (c) the *salience* of the personal disclosure to one's audiences. In the following discussion of each dynamic, it becomes clear that identity modulation is an emergent process between users and technology. This process occurred with previous forms of digital media, but it takes on a particular shape with regard to the platforms and apps examined in this book.

Personal Identifiability

People become personally identifiable when multiple pieces of information about them are aggregated or when a specific piece of information is circulated that conveys one's likeness across contexts or acquaintances. Personal identifiability can be conceived as a spectrum, from complete anonymity to legal, social, and visual recognizability. People self-represent variably along this spectrum in different contexts. For example, in a bank you may present identification with your legal name and a vivid photo of your face, whereas when entering a local coffeeshop you may be known socially to some as their neighbor, but your legal name and other information are left out of this situation. Digital technologies come with features, functionalities, policies, and profit motives that encourage users to self-represent more toward one end of this spectrum or the other. Users also develop norms and etiquette for identifiability. In terms of personal information that identifies us across contexts or to a range of audiences, one's name, face, and location are key pieces of information.

Several scholars have dispelled the notion that early text-based digital technologies enabled complete anonymity and fluid performances of the self (Baym, 2015; Daniels, 2009; Nakamura, 2002). However, many of these technologies allowed individuals to be less personally identifiable through the use of pseudonyms and a lack of photo-sharing functionality. People often took advantage of this to divulge personal information, sharing intimate details that allowed them to form platonic, romantic, and sexual connections. Pseudonyms could even contain provocative and intimate information. Research on gay men's use of the French Minitel—a precursor to the internet—found that their pseudonyms contributed to the eroticization of interactions, indicating physical qualities (e.g., weight, penis size) and location (Livia, 2002). Pseudonyms tightly packed with information resembled the density of newspaper personals (Beauman, 2011), since time on the Minitel was expensive and every character had to count. These men were not completely anonymous in their voluntary sharing of some identifying information, but their lack of personal identifiability regarding legal names and visual semblance allowed for greater freedom in expressing sexual desires. In contrast, a lesbian Minitel community that was focused on political organizing over romantic or sexual interactions compelled members to post using their first names rather than pseudonyms. This expectation of what historian Tamara Chaplin (2014) calls "nominative transparency" (p. 467) was established among users to further their goal of extending offline lesbian communities through the Minitel. While personal identifiability can be rendered more malleable through a technology's features, it is also contingent on norms and expectations that develop with appropriation of these features.

Sentiments regarding "transparency" and "authenticity" in relation to names can also be instilled by technology developers. Facebook provides a well-known example (Raynes-Goldie, 2010), as its early requirement for users to belong to a university or formal organization mandated using a name that was recognizable across these contexts. In public statements, Facebook has associated one's "real" or "authentic" name with transparency. The platform's discursive and programmed requirements for consistent identifiability elide how using a single name across online exchanges facilitates highly profitable data mining and targeted advertising while stymying the management of stigmatized personal information. These requirements pose particularly intensive challenges for LGBTQ people, such as drag queens who wish to self-promote through performer accounts without linking to their nonperformer identities (Lingel & Golub, 2015). Similarly, transgender people may experience difficulties creating a new Facebook account post-transition, since names are often verified through a driver's license or other documents controlled by institutions that often refuse to recognize transgender identities as legitimate (Cavalcante, 2016). Facebook's name policy combines with its features, algorithms, and automated notifications, leading to a situation that anthropologist Alexander Cho (2017) describes as "default publicness." He underscores that default publicness is particularly damaging for marginalized populations, such as queer youth of color, who are often put in socially, emotionally, and economically precarious situations when unintentionally outed through Facebook's design choices.

While text-based digital technologies were not devoid of bodies— physiques, gender expressions, and race all permeated interactions—today's platforms and apps predominantly feature visual media. The functionality for posting photos or videos has become fused with user expectations of being able to see another person's likeness, not just an avatar or symbol. The common practice of taking and posting selfies—using a mobile phone's front-facing camera to capture an image of one's likeness—is often associated with authentic self-representation, since digital photography's accuracy gives the sense that such images are difficult to fake (Tiidenberg, 2018). Since visual self-representation can also serve to affiliate one with a particular group—to self-identify as an insider—it has been an important mode of signaling sexual identity (Frolic, 2001). By including fashion, symbols, or other references to LGBTQ culture, photos have the capacity to replace the words usually associated with coming out. Faces and unique marks on bodies, such as tattoos or birthmarks, make individuals highly identifiable across contexts. But again, unique qualities can be edited or left out of photos, and physical likeness can be communicated without one's face, such as through the "torso pics" that flood Grindr, an app popular with men seeking men.

A person's home or workplace can easily become associated with their name, daily patterns, or other facets of life. Early internet technologies were thought to decouple physical place from digital interactions (Correll, 1995; Quiroz, 2013), but contemporary platforms often incorporate geolocative information automatically. Just like visual appearance, location may be important to signaling sexual identity—indicating arrival at a gay or lesbian venue—or to arranging interactions with other LGBTQ individuals. Geolocative apps can overlay one's sense of physical surroundings and digital interactions, giving rise to what mobile media scholars Larissa Hjorth and Sun Sun Lim (2012) term "mobile intimacy": closeness fostered with others encountered across these blurred public and private boundaries of geographic and electronic space. Studies show that the digital-physical overlay facilitated through mobile applications can help LGBTQ people identify each other, even when physically situated in spaces perceived to be heteronormative (Blackwell et al., 2015; Tang, 2017). Depending on the platform, one may be able to adjust the precision of locational information or obscure their relationship to their current whereabouts. However, the automated processing and display of this information can make it challenging to contain and even dangerous, such as when dating apps are used in countries with laws against homosexuality.

Reach

Many scholars have highlighted the capacity of networked digital technology to broaden the flow of information to vast audiences (Benkler, 2006; Bruns, 2008; Castells, 2009), ushering in an age of "spreadable media" that empowers users to collaboratively create, share, and widely circulate media (Jenkins et al., 2013). Anthropologist Mary L. Gray's (2009) foundational work on the mediated lives of rural queer youth demonstrates the importance of this spreadability. She examines how queer youth who are distant from urban metropolises with larger LGBTQ populations garner representations of LGBTQ identity from media, including websites and social media. As youth develop a sense of sexual identity, digital media also facilitates sharing these identities with select audiences before trying them out in local, physical spaces. Digital media's cross-geographic reach and its affordances for connecting with friendly audiences are pivotal for this identity development. However, the tendency for social media to collapse contexts can also mean that reach is a dynamic to be managed. People may attempt to manage the reach of their personal information by communicating one on one (e.g., through messaging apps), targeting select audiences within a platform, or circulating self-representations of sexual identity across platforms. Concurrently, platforms' affordances and commercial arrangements often facilitate a high level of spreadability across audiences. Through identity modulation, users and platforms shape who sees personal disclosures and how far they spread across networks.

Alongside several scholars (see, e.g., Carrasco & Kerne, 2018; Cassidy, 2018; DeVito et al., 2018; Hanckel et al., 2019; Szulc & Dhoest, 2013), my previous research has focused on how LGBTQ individuals manage the reach of information about their sexual identity (Duguay, 2016a). I have found it useful to think about approaches in terms of what sociologists Jenny Davis and Nathan Jurgenson (2014) have called *context collusions* and *context collisions*. In interviews with LGBTQ university students about their sexual identity disclosures on Facebook, I found that a few made prominent coming-out posts, constituting "context collusions" through which the information was distributed intentionally and expediently across audiences. However, it was more common for individuals to develop strategies for sharing information about sexual identity to some audiences and not others. They expended great effort to avoid "context collusions" wherein information was unintentionally spread across contexts. Similarly, a team of Australian researchers (Hanckel et al., 2019) found that LGBTQ youth employ "identity curation" to manage the boundaries of sharing with family, colleagues, and friends on social media. Youth often posted about sexual identity on platforms unpopulated by the audiences they were not yet out to. In my study (Duguay, 2016a), I similarly found that some participants chose to post more about their sexual identity on platforms like Tumblr, which their parents might not know existed and presumably did not know how to use. Both our studies identified that LGBTQ youth applied stringent criteria for connecting with others, manipulated their content's visibility, and became experts on platforms' privacy features to manage reach.

Algorithms often affect whether and under what circumstances platform audiences see content (Bucher, 2012; Gillespie, 2012). For example, Facebook has tweaked its News Feed algorithm several times, declaring in 2019 that it would prioritize content from friends (presumably over organizations or businesses) based on "signals like how often [users] interact with a given friend, how many mutual friends they have and whether they mark someone as a close friend" (Facebook, 2019). Tinder also serves up the profiles of potential dates based on a special algorithm, which considers user activity and preferences while adjusting to who swipes on your profile (Tinder, 2019). While platform companies give some indications of what their algorithms consider in sorting content, they often remain vague in the name of intellectual property. As Tinder puts it, "We cannot disclose *all* of our secret sauce."

Platforms and apps function in interconnected ways, comprising what media scholars José van Dijck, Thomas Poell, and Martijn de Waal (2018) describe as a "platform ecosystem" (p. 4). They explain how massive "infrastructural platforms," like Amazon or Google, perform the role of gatekeepers who collect and manage flows of data that are valuable to other apps, businesses, and service providers that users access within the platform ecosystem. For example, Tinder allows users to log in through Facebook, an infrastructural platform that has already collected vast amounts of user information, creating a strong informational dependency between these two entities. The bulk of social media activity in the Global North occurs on a limited number of large corporately owned platforms originating within the United States (Nieborg & Poell, 2018; van Dijck et al., 2018).

Media studies scholar Dal Yong Jin (2015) powerfully argues that the concentration of markets, intellectual property, users, and cultural flows into a small number of select platforms gives rise to "platform imperialism," as it "concentrate[s] capital into the hands of a few U.S.-based platform owners, resulting in the expansion of the global divide" (p. 12). Dominant platforms often purchase up-and-coming apps, such as Facebook's acquisition of Instagram and WhatsApp, further concentrating markets and the data collected through these apps. They also deploy spin-off apps to capture a different portion of the market or to offer functionalities apart from their core services, as was the case with Twitter's release of Vine for sharing short videos. This integration among platforms poses hurdles for individuals in treating any single platform as a contained context.

Salience

The final dynamic of identity modulation involves how salient personal disclosures are as self-representations that reflect upon a person's identity. Salience relates to how recognizable this information is to others and, specifically, who recognizes it. This dynamic expands upon Marwick and boyd's (2014) concept of social steganography, a practice in which social media users make posts with certain phrases, images, or other cues in plain sight, banking on only certain members of their audiences possessing the insider knowledge necessary to understand the underlying message. Highly salient self-representations rely on signals of identity that are easily recognizable, whereas less salient self-representations may be vague. In relation to sexual identity, salience can range from, for example, a clear declaration of "I am gay" to a rainbow emoji that is more ambiguous due to its use by allies and other movements.

Media and audiences rely on stereotypes as representations that are recognizable due to their systematic and recurrent presentation across broadcast formats. Communications scholar Ellen Seiter (2017) explains that although stereotypes can be damaging when they suggest that all people within a (perceived, constructed, or self-designated) group are a certain way, they also provide "models of available social identities" (p. 184). Their recurrent images and social norms teach us how to affiliate ourselves with these identities. This logic resonates with assertions that cultural enactments of gender and sexual identity can be learned and performed (Butler, 1990; Plummer, 1996). Learning how to perform a stereotype is what the stars of *RuPaul's Drag Race* (2009–) do when they strut the runway as embellished models of heterosexual femininity.

Stereotypes can function as heuristics for making sense of the world (Lippmann, 1922 cited in Seiter, 2017), enabling audiences to quickly recognize and sort people according to predetermined categories. Even if stereotypes tend to be overgeneralizations, we use them reflexively to reduce our cognitive load and respond to interactional norms. Stereotypical indicators of sexual identity may relate to gender expression, interests, and conduct, such as the stereotype of a lesbian as a masculine, plaid-wearing woman with a knack for fixing things. But stereotypes can change over time. As cultural studies scholar Raymond Williams (1977) observes, new cultural forms often emerge as the recombination of residual understandings with new meanings or knowledge. With media representations of sexual identity diversifying, figure 1.2 describes emergent stereotypes about lesbian and bisexual women, some of which retain masculine traits while adapting to new fashions.

On platforms, salient cultural symbols and stereotypes relating to identity fuse with digital elements. Users appropriate digital technologies in what digital media scholar Jean Burgess (2006) has coined "vernacular creativity," as everyday remediations of cultural resources that become "recognizable because of their familiar elements, and create affective impact through the innovative process of recombination" (p. 206). As people participate in vernacular creativity, they demonstrate digital skills alongside insider knowledge of the cultural signals being mobilized, which constitute not only popular cultural knowledge but also an understanding of platform cultures. Being adept in digital culture has become so integral to engaging with others that scholars have begun reconceptualizing digital literacy in light of this (Gleason, 2018; Kanai, 2016; Wargo, 2015). Being digitally

---

lesbian & bi girl style is like:

- **denim on denim**
- **tank top. shorts. sandals. done.**
- **the most wildly extravagant shit u can think of, but dug out of a bargain bin**
- **intentionally clashing patterns**
- **goth but sort of lazy about it**
- **barbecue dad but make it slutty**

93,361 notes | 6:17pm 3 Jul 2019 Tagged: #this is an abridged selection i could not hope to write a comprehensive guide #personally i am lazy goth and discount extravagance in cold weather #and slutty bbq dad all summer

Figure 1.2 Tumblr user post discussing recognizable fashion trends among lesbian and bisexual women, July 3, 2019. Source: https://chthonicillness.tumblr.com/post/18603 4735896.

literate means not only being able to use the latest technologies but also being able to understand and participate in the norms and practices of emergent digital cultures.

Tailoring identity-related content so that it becomes salient to desired social media audiences therefore involves both conventional indicators of identity and elements of digital culture. If we understand digital culture to involve technological affordances and the cultures of use that emerge from their appropriation, digital culture can assume a wide array of forms. Memes, emoji, and hashtags are some of the most prominent elements of digital culture featured throughout this book. Memes are representations that users share and creatively build on in ways that establish boundaries between in-groups, who understand the message or joke, and out-groups, who may not get the joke or may even be its target (Miltner, 2018). For example, some Pride-related memes use image macro templates to critique corporations for their commercial co-optation of these celebrations (Dockray, 2019). They draw boundaries between queer activists and corporate entities, many of whom miss the critique if they do not recognize the memetic format or take it seriously as a cultural expression. Hashtags also combine digital functionality—the # that hyperlinks and categorizes content—with user-created expressions. While hashtags can gather users in dialogue about a particular topic or help to form communities (Bruns & Burgess, 2015), they can also be reflective of individual identity (Highfield & Leaver, 2015). This will become apparent in later analysis of Instagram and Vine hashtags.

Emoji differ from these other elements of digital culture due to limited user control over their visual design. While originating as user-generated keyboard punctuation, emoji have been incorporated into Unicode Standard format, which is an international specification for character sets across hardware and software (Unicode Inc., 2019). Unicode Standard was developed, and is maintained, by the Unicode Consortium, a nonprofit organization comprised of technology corporations (e.g., Apple, Google, Facebook), governments, researchers, and other donors. Communications scholars Luke Stark and Kate Crawford (2015) describe how emoji are centralized through the Unicode Standard but differentiated in their design through platform and device-specific fonts, which remain corporate intellectual property. While users interpret emoji in multiple ways, Stark and Crawford argue that emoji generate "information capital" (p. 8) for platforms as they instrumentalize and standardize affect—the emotions and sentiments that emoji convey—to render it into trackable, monetizable data.

This standardization includes the replication of stereotypes through emoji. The Unicode emoji "two women holding hands" (🏳️‍🌈) appears often in self-representations throughout this book, providing an apt example of gender stereotypes that become "baked in" to technological designs (Bivens & Haimson, 2016). While many queer women whom I interviewed adopted this emoji as shorthand for same-gender attraction, it does not reflect these women's diversity. Across platforms, its figures display feminine haircuts and clothing (e.g., skirts). They appear with a yellow skin tone by default, while other skin tones were only added with subsequent updates (Miltner, 2020). Sometimes the women are even identical, as in Facebook's version, precluding their use to indicate attraction to another woman. In light of these options, Mozilla's depiction appears to be the most progressive, since it includes a short-haired woman who is also wearing pants—revolutionary!

Emoji provide insight into just one of many ways that platforms shape the salience of self-representations conveying personal information. Some aesthetics, behaviors, or self-expressions may be more common on certain platforms, stemming from a "platform vernacular" (Gibbs et al., 2016) that interweaves affordances and user practices in a "unique combination of styles, grammars, and logics" (p. 257). The salience of sexual identity disclosures may become lost within a platform vernacular, such as how Pride selfies posted to Instagram may be interpreted as showing off the festival's aesthetics in response to the platform's visual emphasis rather than making a personal statement. On the other hand, self-representations of sexual identity may become part of the platform vernacular, like YouTube's burgeoning genre of "coming out" videos (Alexander & Losh, 2010). While these are highly salient expressions, leaving little ambiguity in their messages, their popularity may also draw questions about authenticity, individuality, and whether one is just joining in for the attention (Cunningham & Craig, 2019).

Overall, the salience of personal disclosures on social media depend on individuals' self-representations, the cultural and digital literacy of their audiences, and platforms' cultures of use and affordances. In referring to "affordances" throughout this book, I invoke ecological and design understandings of what artifacts or technologies enable people to do (Gibson, 1979; Norman, 1988), with "constraints" as a shorthand for the opposite of affordances. I also have in mind updates to the concept regarding digital media technologies, which view affordances as stemming from users' everyday practices; the combined layers of hardware, operating system/interface, and apps on a device; and the complex and ever-changing relationship between platforms and users (Bucher & Helmond, 2017; McVeigh-Schultz & Baym, 2015). Communications scholars Peter Nagy and Gina Neff (2015) describe "imagined affordances" as those that "evoke the imagination of both users and designers" (p. 1)—these individuals may not be fully aware of their expectations or anticipated uses of technologies, but such imaginings become instantiated in a technology's actual design and use. The authors' elaborated definition highlights three aspects that I view as pivotal: "Imagined affordances emerge between *users'* perceptions, attitudes, and expectations; between the *materiality* and functionality of technologies; and between the intentions and perceptions of *designers*" (p. 5, emphasis added). A platform's user population, the materiality of its technological architecture (i.e., its stuff—features, functions, buttons, devices), and its designers, including developers and business owners, all contribute to the imagined affordances that affect how the platform features in the sharing and reception of personal disclosures.

A Framework for Identity Modulation

Identity modulation is the process by which these dynamics become modified and adjusted, or modulated, when individuals share personal disclosures on social media. Both the user and the platform play a role in the degree of personal identifiability, reach, and salience of information shared as it circulates through networked technology and (potentially) across audiences from multiple social contexts. Figure 1.3 gives a sense of the extent to which these dynamics can be modulated: personal identifiability can range from anonymity to full legal, social, and visual identifiability; reach can span from one-on-one interactions to one-to-many formats across audiences within the same platform or across platforms; and salience can vary from ambiguity and unnoticeability to an absolutely clear declaration of identity that is widely recognizable. However, this is a general illustration, as the degrees of each dynamic are relative to the context and situation. For example, one's face may not be personally identifying

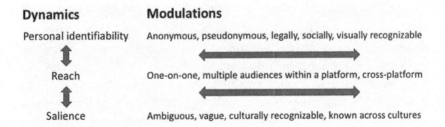

Dynamics

Personal identifiability

Reach

Salience

Modulations

Anonymous, pseudonymous, legally, socially, visually recognizable

One-on-one, multiple audiences within a platform, cross-platform

Ambiguous, vague, culturally recognizable, known across cultures

Figure 1.3 Identity modulation framework.
Source: Illustration by author

when used in a dating app profile while traveling in the same way that it would be when using the app in one's small hometown.

Identity modulation's dynamics are often adjusted in relation to each other. One might be apt to include details that increase personal identifiability if a self-representation's reach is limited. In turn, if a personal disclosure's salience is low, and only certain audiences will *get* how it reflects on the individual, then one might choose to extend its reach by making the post public. However, platforms often default toward compiling users' information to heighten their identifiability and extending the reach of user activity in the name of sharing.

I have previously worked with the ideas of reach and salience in considering the impact of sexual identity representations on social media (Duguay, 2016b). Examining representations of Ruby Rose, an LGBTQ celebrity, I theorized about the capacity for a self-representation to garner engagement. When could Rose's social media posts make a statement or inspire others to share about their sexual identity? I drew on the work of media scholar Anastasia Kavada (2015), who asserts, "Conversations are what social media are designed for and where they draw their power from" (p. 1). She underscores that although platforms are now the "architects of conversations," as developers and administrators of these networked technologies, users can also find empowerment in the conversations they spark. Some of Ruby Rose's social media posts were strikingly salient in their queerness, lending themselves to powerful conversations in fan responses and media coverage, while others appeared to be absorbed in Instagram's platform vernacular of glamorous photos.

Situating these ideas within the framework of identity modulation allows me to extend and move beyond discussions of LGBTQ visibility and media representation. Sometimes discussions of visibility focus on what is or is not there. Indeed, this is important, since minorities missing from view cannot be acknowledged, let alone attempt to rupture the dominant structures that invisibilize them. Across many countries and online, media visibility in this sense is no longer a problem for LGBTQ people. In fact, communication scholar Kevin Barnhust (2007) observed that the proliferation of queer visibility is a double-edged sword: with greater visibility comes the potential for commercialization and assimilation that risks "converting radicalism into a market niche" (p. 1). As such, many pivotal critiques of LGBTQ media visibility highlight its commercialized and homonormative qualities (Gross, 2001; Ng, 2013). Moving from broader media representation to self-representation through contemporary digital media, investigating individuals, their connections, and the technologies they use warrants a different lens for analysis. Identity modulation and its dynamics allow for a granular examination of what is happening when individuals make their sexual identity visible through social media— what they do, how they manage it, and to what degree it is visible—understanding visibility not as a binary but a spectrum. Further, identity modulation makes space for examining the role of social media platforms as co-arbiters of visibility through their affordances, politics, economic interests, and cultures of use.

Given this multifaceted approach to understanding personal disclosure, this framework proposes a departure from the notion of visibility,[5] and its association with what can be seen, toward an auditory metaphor of modulation that elucidates identity negotiations between individuals and platforms. Through this research, I have noticed that the impact of personal disclosures made through social media come not merely from their visibility but from their contributions to pivotal conversations. To attain this, individuals need to have a sense of agency in modulating their disclosures. People must possess an ability to adjust their degree of personal identifiability, the reach of their content, and the salience of their personal disclosures in order to invoke such outcomes. They need to be heard, in their own voice and by those they want to hear them. Many examples throughout these chapters illustrate the tension that occurs when platforms complicate or refuse individuals' attempts at identity modulation. These instances open up possibilities for imagining the radical outcomes that may be realized in a world where social media truly empower people to express themselves as digital citizens.

METHODS AND IDENTITIES IN THE MIDDLE

Similar to how signal processing happens in the "middle of media" (Sterne & Rodgers, 2011, p. 35), identity modulation occurs in the middle of digital self-representation. Tackling its apparent seamlessness requires a research approach in the middle of bodies of knowledge, methods, and aspects of identity. This book is situated within the multidisciplinary fields of internet studies and digital media studies while drawing from scholarly studies of media, literature, sociology, sexuality, gender, and race. My research adopted mixed methods combining traditional interview and textual analysis approaches with digital methods, as ways of examining "born digital" artifacts (Berry, 2011), from individual posts to entire platforms. I also scoped this research around queer women's self-representations, understanding queer women to be often in the middle—or forgotten—in terms of research, LGBTQ issues, and identity.

Breaking apart the seamlessness of digital self-representation required research methods examining the constitutive role of platforms, users, and social media content, which I expand on in the appendix. With Ben Light and Jean Burgess, I developed a systematic approach for analyzing apps called the "walkthrough method" (Light et al., 2018). This method enables the researcher to identify how an app guides users and shapes self-representations through its affordances and embedded cultural references. While we wrote about the method specifically in relation to apps (i.e., smartphone applications), I use this term interchangeably with "platform," referring to services that provide technological scaffolding as well as governing and economic oversight for digitally mediated participation. The services examined in this research are predominantly engaged with as apps, offering reduced functionality through desktop versions. I applied the walkthrough method to Tinder, Instagram, and Vine, three apps with a volume of content created and circulated by queer women in 2014–17 when I conducted this research.

The internet's vast troves of queer content certainly posed challenges for choosing particular apps to focus on. However, these apps stood out as situating queer women's activity within their broader mainstream uptake, necessitating the negotiation of self-representations in relation to the mix of users who may intercept them. In contrast to LGBTQ-specific apps, they also present features and functionalities that were not necessarily developed with queer users in mind. In addition to this rationale, I was already on these apps, noticing the concentration in queer women's activity that was largely absent from other spaces in my life. As a dating app largely marketed toward heterosexual users, Tinder caught my attention for the range of profiles created by women seeking women. Instagram, a predominantly photo-based app that later added video functionality, was exploding with queer content and controversy, as LGBTQ celebrities increasingly signed on, while users called for less censorship of women's bodies, such as through the expanding #freethenipple campaign. Vine was an overwhelming sensory experience with many similarities to a more contemporary video-based app, TikTok (a connection I return to in the book's conclusion). Released in 2013, three years following Instagram's debut, Vine's affordances for anonymity, lesser-known status, and relaxed policies attracted youth and users looking for a different experience. As Vines—the short looping videos people created—were easily embedded across other platforms and websites, the app's user base grew rapidly (Bennett, 2013). While rumors of platforms becoming defunct are sometimes treated as the horror stories of digital media studies, threatening to render research obsolete, I feel fortunate to have immersed myself in queer female

Viners' content while the app was thriving. Their activity, along with my observations of Vine's promotional materials, policies, and updates, allowed for building an archive that could no longer be pieced together due to the app's discontinuation and fragmentation of any remaining content. This archive demonstrates the app's vibrant queer exchanges, its users' creativity, and its opportunities and constraints for self-representation. These findings only gain relevance as new and existing apps integrate similar affordances, especially relating to short videos, and see comparable uses.

My experiences on these apps spurred me to turn a research lens on them, combining walkthrough materials with analysis of queer women's content and experiences. I used digital tools (when available) and applied textual and visual analysis (McKee, 2003; Rose, 2012) to examine content tagged with queer women's hashtags across Instagram and Vine, as well as Tinder profiles gathered with consent. I supplemented this analysis with the experiences, opinions, insights, and aims of queer women whom I interviewed about their self-representation on these platforms. Gathering participants from LGBTQ networks and directly through these apps, I interviewed ten Tinder users, eight Instagrammers, and two Viners from across several countries and subject positions. This combined analysis, involving close investigation of apps, hundreds of social media posts, and twenty interviews, provides the basis for this book's theory building around identity modulation. Although social media technologies and their uses are always changing, alongside shifts in meanings and symbols attached to sexual identity, this research aims toward theoretical transferability to provide insights into future configurations of people and technology.

While I have outlined how a focus on sexual identity brings to light processes of identity modulation, there is an urgency to studying LGBTQ self-representation, especially queer women's self-representation. Across many countries, LGBTQ people have attained protection from harassment and murder and, to a lesser extent, established the right to adopt children and have their relationships legally recognized (Nunez, 2016). While working on this project, history was made when the Australian parliament voted in favor of recognizing same-sex marriage in 2017. However, this decision was only reached after a nonbinding postal survey, inviting the entire population to weigh in on the rights of a minority. Months of heated discussion, worry, and publicly broadcasted lobbying that demonized homosexuality took a toll on LGBTQ communities, instilling fear, sorrow, and weariness (Hunt, 2018). I witnessed the stress of this uncertainty firsthand, seeing the toll it took on my partner as she waited and wondered if her family members would vote yes.

The politics of countries where I have resided have taught me that the myths of "progress" are that it is linear and has an endpoint. Yes, Australia has legalized same-sex marriage, but there have been multiple physical assaults against attendees at Sydney's Gay and Lesbian Mardi Gras, the country's largest Pride festival, in subsequent years (Dias, 2019). Yes, Canada introduced a commemorative coin boasting about equality (Harris, 2019), but Black Lives Matter activists highlight the continued profiling and police brutality against racialized queer and transgender people (Walcott, 2017). These fluctuations echo elsewhere and reinforce the stigmatization of nonheterosexual and noncisgender identities with grave impacts on people's lives.

My least favorite part of researching sexual identity is dredging up evidence of just how pressingly we need to pay attention to the well-being, social connections, and experiences of LGBTQ people. Such research articles are often similar, as studies of sexual minorities from clinical, psychological, and health perspectives, and they are heartbreaking, since they show that LGBTQ people generally experience high rates of physical and mental health problems and are at higher risk of suicide than heterosexual, cisgender populations (Almeida et al., 2009; Goldblum et al., 2012; Gonzales et al., 2016; Haas et al., 2010; Lytle et al., 2014). Regarding queer women, studies show that they experience higher rates of mental health problems than heterosexual women (Colledge et al., 2015; Kerr et al., 2013). Bisexual and transgender women in particular experience high rates of distress, discrimination, and mental health issues (Leonard et al., 2015; Watson et al., 2018). Scholars refute the narrow, but surprisingly still common, thinking that an individual's identification as LGBTQ *causes* these problems (Valdiserri et al., 2019). Instead, they underscore how enduring stigma against LGBTQ people creates stressful circumstances, such as family rejection or bullying, which can negatively impact mental health. Yes, some aspects of life have changed for LGBTQ people, especially in countries where their human rights are legally recognized, but there is no endpoint in sight in terms of the need to continue addressing these inequalities.

Despite this urgency, there is still a tangible lack of research about queer women across fields and especially within digital media studies. In the 1990s, literary scholar Terry Castle (1993) argued that the "lesbian" was an apparitional figure, barely noticeable across politics, media, and literature and overshadowed by gay men, subsumed by queer theory's focus on male homosexuality. Luckily, there are now several brilliant scholars researching queer women's media representation and indeed a handful researching queer women's digital media, whom I cite frequently. However, there is still an apparitional quality to this topic. Several foundational studies of sexuality and early digital media focus on gay men's chat rooms and discussion forums (Campbell, 2004; McGlotten, 2013; Mowlabocus, 2010), while mobile media's uptake has been matched by burgeoning literature about gay men's apps and social networks (Ahlm, 2016; Blackwell et al., 2015; Brubaker et al., 2016; Gudelunas, 2012; Licoppe et al., 2016; Roth, 2015). Several studies of LGBTQ people also lump us together, yielding findings unspecific to queer women. To help address this scholarly disparity, I provide a vivid account of queer women's digital self-representation, recognizing their experiences in their own right as well as what they can tell us more broadly about personal disclosures on social media.

Lastly, queer women—as the term implies—live within the intersection of sexual identity with a gender identity (female) that is often subject to systemic bias, alongside other elements of identity that may heighten experiences of discrimination and inequality. Black feminists stress the importance of addressing multiple forms of oppression, such as racism, sexism, and class injustice, which individuals experience in relation to overlapping identity positions (Combahee River Collective, 1986; Crenshaw, 1991). I take care to note how individuals' specific positionality matters for their identity modulation. Individual differences also combine with shared identifications, such as the shared experiences of women in this book as nonheterosexual and female, which sometimes put them at the crossroads of heterosexism and sexism or misogyny. Feminist efforts to counter gender inequalities have been subject to intense backlash, often occurring online, in the form of increasing attacks and harassment by "men's rights" and antifeminist groups (Marwick & Lewis, 2017; Phillips, 2015). In identity modulation, personal information about one aspect of identity is often modulated in relation to other aspects of identity. Adjustments to one's personal identifiability or the reach of a self-representation may be made not only with indications of sexual identity in mind but also in light of how audiences will respond to coinciding expressions of gender or race. This is a pertinent time to focus on how queer women approach identity modulation, since their everyday experiences of social media are inextricably related to their personal self-representation while being situated within broader societal developments.

WHAT IDENTITY MODULATION DOES

The chapters that follow present a close analysis of the processes of identity modulation, in turn focusing on how platforms and individuals negotiate the dynamics of personal identifiability, reach, and salience. The next chapter centers the negotiation of personal identifiability, as queer women respond to Tinder's importing of highly personally identifiable information from Facebook as a means for generating profiles intended to attest to others' trustworthiness. Queer women I spoke with found that these platform-generated identities were conducive to attempts at deception and misrepresentation by heterosexual men, women, and couples. They tended to increase the salience of sexual identity in their profiles to deter these users while signaling their intention to date other queer women, managing their reach and personal identifiability in light of this heightened salience. Their repeated and often stereotyped signaling of sexual identity gave rise to what Lindsay Ferris and I (2019) have termed a lesbian digital imaginary: the fusion of cultural and digital references to identity that are imagined to resonate with a shared community. While the lesbian digital imaginary drew some boundaries of exclusion, requiring individuals to demonstrate a particular cultural and digital literacy, it also enabled several women to connect and build trustworthiness as they added other modes of communication allowing for intimate, reliable self-representation.

Chapters 3 and 4 shift from Tinder's one-on-one exchanges to Instagram and Vine as public-facing platforms necessitating the negotiation of vast audiences. Chapter 3 focuses on reach, as it examines processes of identity modulation in queer women's self-branding. Instagram's filters and their association with hip and glamorous aesthetics, as well as Vine's 6.5-second looping video, combine with other digital affordances of these apps to provide users with the capacity to draw attention from others, heightening their reach by gathering a following. The queer women I interviewed responded to these affordances by modulating their reach in relation to salience through labor that integrated sexual identity into self-branding to support their day jobs, side gigs, or hobbies. These forms of labor included *intimate affective*, formulating relatable personal disclosures that convey intimate details; *developmental aesthetic*, the effort expended in acquiring and practicing skills necessary to create a persona or appearance that resonates with one's target audience; and *aspiring relational*, putting shared identity to work in attempts to build relationships with those who already have large followings. As these women enacted this labor, their production of personal and creative content gave rise to feelings of exploitation and alienation alongside opportunities for greater social and economic participation.

Chapter 4 looks at queer women's self-representation on Instagram and Vine from a different angle, uncovering how varying degrees of salience relating to sexual identity can give rise to particular kinds of publics and counterpublics. I highlight the prominent representations of normatively feminine, white, slim, and glamorous women and lifestyles on queer women's Instagram hashtags as reflective of a networked intimate public that can provide a sense of community but remains fairly apolitical. This networked intimate public gives the impression that the "good life" of neoliberal citizenship is now attainable for those queer women who are able to perpetuate homonormative appearances. In contrast, queer women's circulation of highly salient representations of sexual identity on Vine in the form of thirst traps, intimate expressions, and counternormative discourse facilitated the formation of counterpublics. These counterpublics often circulated challenges to heterosexism, racism, and other forms of oppression, which were sometimes made visible through the platform's trending feature. However, the salience of these women's sexual identity made them targets for censorship, harassment, and discrimination on both Instagram and Vine. Platforms' policies and moderation processes failed to protect them, providing a patchwork of governing mechanisms insufficient to address populations of users who harness platform affordances to antagonize others.

With these chapters illustrating how, when individuals are able to steer it, identity modulation can contribute to the formation of relationships, greater social and economic participation, and discourses that challenge the status quo, the concluding chapter asserts the need for individuals to have greater agency over these processes. I analyze the hurdles that queer women encountered in their identity modulation, which implicate platforms' infrastructures, business models, and governance approaches as well as broader social, political, and economic influences. The narrow boundaries of digital imaginaries, the capacity for individuals to experience exploitation and undercompensation for their productive labor, and the patchwork platform governance that enables targeting vulnerable users are all complex problems for identity modulation. I propose that although there is not one simple solution, these issues can be addressed at multiple levels of platform design and economic arrangements, as well as through platforms taking responsibility for the cultures of use that thrive thanks to their policies and affordances. Given that identity modulation is not only applicable in the management of information about sexual identity but also integral to restoring context for intimate and personal disclosures on social media, I assert that identity modulation must be protected as a right within individuals' digital citizenship.

CHAPTER 2

Queering Tinderella

Personal Identifiability in Platform-Generated Identities

"Do you think true love could ever be found through Tinder?" Journalists often wrap up with broad and polarizing questions, and this particular interview was no different. This query followed thirty minutes of critical discussion about the mobile app's design and functionality.

"Yes, sure, I met my partner on there." My response brought the interview to a standstill, and before I could clarify, the reporter thanked me for my time and hung up. I watched the newspaper in the subsequent days, but the story never ran. I told myself that stories are often cut depending on editorial whims or breaking news. But it was also possible that my final statement had complicated the narrative too much. I had raised points about how Tinder automated the creation of profiles, generating identities on behalf of users in ways that affected their self-representation, and yet my experience reflected that the app could indeed still play a role in helping people form relationships. And it was not just my experience; I have interviewed several queer women who met friends and partners through Tinder. However, the journalist had not let me paint the full picture: it was not as easy as the swipe of a thumb. Partner seeking on Tinder required queer women to work at identity modulation, in large part to resist the app's automated representation of users.

Initially, creating an account on Tinder is quick. It requires only the tap of a button if you already have a Facebook account. However, thinking back to when I signed up in late 2014, I recall taking additional steps. Although the app brought me directly to a screen where I could browse others'

Personal but Not Private. Stefanie Duguay, Oxford University Press. © Oxford University Press 2022.
DOI: 10.1093/oso/9780190076184.003.0002

profiles, I immediately went to my own profile and started to edit the default information imported from Facebook. I wrote a short bio about being an international student from Canada working on my PhD in Australia and drinking a lot of coffee, throwing in emoji where appropriate. Then I curated my photos, including one posing with a kangaroo to back up my self-description, since apparently this is not something locals are prone to do (see figure 2.1). Despite having changed my Facebook settings to "interested in" both men and women following my subtle coming-out post years earlier, Tinder had placed me in the default category of seeking men, which I changed to seeking women.

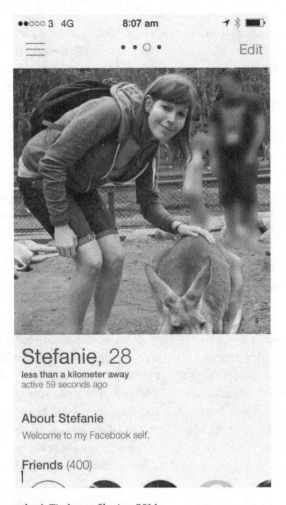

Figure 2.1 The author's Tinder profile circa 2014.

Finally, I thought I was ready to start swiping. However, in the browse screen I found myself staring at others' profiles, trying to discern their intentions: Why was this person on the app? Who were they looking for? While Tinder's profile-sorting algorithm served up many users in my densely populated neighborhood, I hesitated to swipe right on anyone. Several women appeared to pose flirtatiously with men in their photos and declared they were looking for "just friends." Other profiles seemed to belong to men or displayed poorly photoshopped supermodels. It was not long before I had left swiped (dismissed) everyone in my vicinity and was met with a pulsating message: "There's no one new around you!" One of my interview participants would later sadly describe this as reaching "the end of Tinder," where either you must change your settings or move locations, or those around you must change.

In the end, I only went on one Tinder date. I matched with her one day while waiting for the bus. I opened with "Happy Monday!," and she thought it was utterly strange that someone would start with such a salutation. I backpedaled, describing how the sun was beautifully filtering onto the bus stop and feeling at a loss to describe the contrast with Canada's December weather. After I arrived at work, our conversation was put on hiatus until the end of the day, when she messaged that she was eating strawberries, followed by three enthusiastic strawberry emoji: 🍓 🍓 🍓. It was my turn to think this person was a bit odd. I flicked through her photos once more, which consecutively showed her in a cycling jersey, in a fancy dress, with a new tattoo, and bungee jumping. The contrast was huge, and there was no way to place them in chronological order. Still, we set up a coffee date for a few days later and exchanged phone numbers, texting to get to know each other a bit and to open a more immediate line of communication if one of us had to cancel.

On the day of the date, I woke up with a hearty skepticism, found an acceptable outfit with my roommate's help, and let him know which café we were meeting at in case I needed rescuing. Thanks to Tinder's importing of Facebook information, I knew this person's "authentic" name, age, and interests, as well as whether or not we had friends in common (we did not). I had a sense of what she might look like but was not sure which variation was the latest. I also knew a few details from our text conversations, but I had no way of verifying any of them. I had so much personally identifying information about this individual, yet I only started really getting to know who she was during that first date and in the subsequent weeks, months, and years.

Tinder presents a peculiar context for identity modulation. Personal identifiability is high by default due to the app's previous requirement—and residual expectation—that users sign in through Facebook. However, the reach of personal information is constrained by proximity: you only see individuals within a specified radius of your smartphone (up to 160 km/ 100 mi. on the free version). Since Tinder's features are organized around this imported information and, more focally, the profile photos that fill its swipe screen, other identity-related information is less salient. Even if users share more in the biography field or in messages, this information appears less tangible than that which has been imported from Facebook. Tinder's high level of personal identifiability and low salience point to why I felt I knew very little about my coffee date but still had some confidence she would resemble her profile when I met her in person.

Further, profiles are generated within the context of an app that has been marketed, and embraced in the media, as a staple of heterosexual hook-up culture. A video from the comedy website College Humor (2014) entitled *Tinderella: A Modern Fairy Tale* reflects the app's popular reputation. It plays on Disney's animated film with a cartoon featuring Cindy, short for Cinderella, swiping left on every Tinder profile save for that of Princeton, a handsome prince charming who courts her with "Sup?" after they match. Shortly after meeting at The Ball, a local bar, the next scene shows them under the covers of Princeton's bed, with sex implied through squeaking noises. While Princeton is still sleeping, Cindy quietly leaves in the morning as the narrator announces, "They lived happily ever after because they never spoke again."

In stark contrast to the original Cinderella's focus on finding one true love, modern-day Tinderella and her suitors are intent on casual sexual encounters, which are depicted as being devoid of romance or long-term potential. As media scholar Kath Albury (2018) observes, Tinder has become embroiled in the longstanding scandalization and disparagement of heterosexual casual sex in contrast to sex within marriage or long-term relationships. She argues that Tinder's gamification through the swipe implicates it within the "game" of casual sex, which functions according to rules based on heterosexual gender scripts that call on women to be sexually liberated while simultaneously risking being shamed as "too slutty." These scripts also reward men reputationally for sexual behavior without similar threats of shame. Despite some efforts by the company to promote Tinder as a tool for "social discovery" (Craw, 2014), intended for a range of social purposes, it became known as a hook-up app for heterosexual partner seekers. As I swiped through multitudes of women's profiles displaying clubwear and copious amounts of makeup, I could not help but feel I had stumbled into a game where I was not playing on either team. And indeed, it reminded me of being at a straight nightclub. That is, until I started finding other ways of recognizing queer women on the app.

This chapter examines how Tinder's affordances and cultures of use give rise to its identity modulation dynamics by centering platform-generated user identities, which are framed within perceptions of Tinder as a heteronormative hook-up app. Analysis of the app is paired with interviews conducted in 2016 with ten queer female users hailing from Australia and Canada. Drawing from interview participants' experiences, it is easy to see how platform-generated identities actually facilitate deception by making it seem as though this default information is a sufficient indicator of trustworthiness. In response, many of the queer women I spoke with chose to enhance the salience of their sexual identity on Tinder as a way of attracting other queer women and weeding out users who were not queer women but still appeared in their searches. With this heightened salience, several individuals also felt the need to manage the reach and personal identifiability of their profiles, since Tinder's use in certain physical contexts could out them, and their sexual or romantic desires, to unintended audiences. Overall, this chapter illustrates how an app can play a large role in its users' representation while placing such representations within a heteronormative framing that warrants responsive and resistant actions on the part of queer women to identify and build trust with each other as the foundation for sparking relationships.

PREPOPULATING IDENTITIES

In a 2013 journal article, three computer scientists turned their attention to online dating, noting that dating apps raised concerns about the trustworthiness of potential dates (Norcie et al., 2013). They set up an experimental interface that incorporated social media information into dating profiles and recruited 161 people through Amazon's clickwork platform Mechanical Turk to record the new interface's impact on their worries about misrepresentation in dating profiles. Respondents reported a decrease in concerns, leading the researchers to conclude that they had successfully "bootstrapped trust" into online dating. *Bootstrap* is a common computer science term that describes loading software into a system or program. When a computer "boots" up, it loads the operating system into its memory, which sets all other tasks on their way. The researchers argued that loading social media data into a dating app enabled identity verification, thus transferring trust into the dating system, allowing daters to match with each other worry free.

Although these researchers were a little late to be describing Tinder, which launched in 2012, the idea that importing social media data imparts trust into a system is useful for understanding Tinder's premise. The app was developed in a start-up incubator owned by InterActiveCorp (IAC), the American holding company responsible for the formation of Match Group, a conglomerate of dating sites and apps that includes, for example, Plenty of Fish and OkCupid (Shontell, 2014). However, dating through digital means was not yet as popular as it would later become, with 30 percent of American adults having used a dating website or app by 2020 (Anderson et al., 2020). Despite online dating's promise to open the door to a global pool of dates, many people were deterred by the perceived risk of meeting "strangers" on the internet and the possibility for others to misrepresent themselves in dating profiles (Anderson, 2005; Gibbs et al., 2011). With the introduction of mobile dating apps, users became (re)anchored in physical space through features displaying potential suitors in relation to their proximity. This geolocational functionality generates what mobile communications scholar Adriana de Souza e Silva (2006) refers to as "hybrid space" that "merges the borders between physical and digital spaces" (p. 265). Due to gay men's use of earlier digital technologies to arrange physical encounters, this population became early adopters of dating apps (Gudelunas, 2012). However, the apps' entry into mainstream dating practices was slower due to existing stigma and safety concerns, primarily held by women because of the responsibility placed on them to avoid and deflect sexually aggressive or violent situations (Farvid & Aisher, 2016).

On top of these hesitations, Tinder's main user-sorting functionality—the swipe—necessitates greater reassurance that users can trust the people they match with and, in turn, trust the app. Profile browsing takes the form of a repeated swipe gesture: left for "no" and right to "like" another person. Swipes are based primarily on profile photos, which dominate the screen in browse mode, accompanied by little other information. The flow of swiping must be paused to view a user's self-composed biography, among other information, by tapping the screen and navigating through a profile in detail. Jokes about getting "Tinder thumb" from swiping too much and laments about mindless swiping indicate that this gesture is the norm rather than scrutinizing full profiles (Brock, 2014; Vine, 2018). Tinder cofounder and former CEO Sean Rad has described the app's main activity of swiping as a game (Stampler, 2014), and its design harks back to rating websites like Hot or Not and Facebook's initial iteration Facemash, which allowed Harvard students to rank each other (Kaplan, 2003). Visual media scholars Gaby David and Carolina Cambre (2016) discuss these design choices as instantiating a "swipe logic" of rapid, binary decision-making encouraged through "built-in psychologically persuasive patterning" (p. 7). These qualities of the swipe make it difficult to regard as a gesture reflecting concerted evaluation of potential partners, or even as intentional as buying someone a drink at a bar to get to know them better.

Even so, when two people swipe right on each other, Tinder presents a jovial match screen and enables sending text-based messages. In an interview, Rad explained the swipe's double opt-in system through a primitive mating metaphor. He stated, "If you're a hunter, there's constant rejection. And if you're hunted, you're constantly being bombarded" (Lapowsky, n.d.). Since Tinder only notifies users of mutual interest, this avoids the risk of rejection and lets the "hunted" people feel less overwhelmed. Although this may be the case, downloading an app that enables rapidly being *hunted* by others who know your approximate location still seems like a tough sell.

Enter the notion of bootstrapping trust. For years, as Tinder's popularity grew, the app required users to log in through Facebook. This single sign-on functionality was already common, as Google and Facebook offered verification across many web services, enabling users to cut down on creating new accounts and passwords. Tinder took this one step further, creating not only an account but a user's dating profile from available Facebook information, including one's name, age, gender, recent photos, interests (i.e., pages liked), and friend network. As mentioned in chapter 1, Facebook's policy wording has changed over the years, but the platform has always urged individuals to use their legal names, with current disputes over "authentic identities" being resolved by users providing legal documents, such as a driver's license. Scholars have also found that the propensity for people to Facebook "friend" those already known to them results in users generally striving to give self-presentations consistent with existing impressions (Baym, 2015; Lim et al., 2012; Zhao et al., 2008). Along with this, people post to Facebook and add friends over time, accumulating an archive of their lives (Robards & Lincoln, 2017). Although some users put joke responses and refuse to complete profile fields, a fairly accurate Facebook profile conveys a high level of personal identifiability in Tinder due to the display of one's legal or socially recognizable name paired with photos vetted by Facebook friends and GPS information. Tinder has espoused this high personal identifiability to allay user concerns about matches, declaring in the app's 2014 FAQs (now removed): "We use Facebook to make sure you are matched with real people who share similar interests and common friends." Therefore, realness and, in turn, trustworthiness on Tinder equate to having a Facebook account.

This logic is inevitably flawed. Anyone with an email address or mobile number can create a Facebook account and link it to Tinder. Furthermore, data that Tinder imports do not indicate whether a potential match has a difficult-to-fake Facebook account of posts accumulated over time or an account created recently with just enough information to fulfill Tinder's demands. More pertinent to this book's overarching concerns, the imported information does not necessarily involve the level of personal disclosure that may be important in intimate, sexual, and romantic contexts. Relationship status and sexual preferences constitute information that is likely to seem out of place on Facebook, depending on the audiences one has amassed there. However, people who are dating or hooking up must often determine their compatibility through these basic details. I have argued elsewhere that Facebook, as a platform requiring meticulous impression management due to overlapping audiences, encourages normative displays of identity (Duguay, 2017). This echoes sociologist Bernie Hogan's (2010) assertion that the accumulation of overlapping audiences on Facebook spurs identity performances tailored to the *"lowest common denominator* of what is normatively acceptable" (p. 383) to these audiences.

By incorporating Facebook as the measure of trustworthiness, Tinder encourages users to import these normative standards into its app, with profiles that do not seem Facebook friendly appearing out of place. Among men seeking men, Tinder is known as the less sexualized alternative to gay dating apps, the app to which men turn when looking for "nice guys" (MacKee, 2016). Thus, Tinder's importing of socially surveilled self-representations from Facebook has given rise to a predominantly vanilla dating app for gay men. For users in general, the lack of default information about sexuality, desires, and sexual identity appears to uphold the company's aspiration to be known for catalyzing weddings and long-term relationships while downplaying its use to initiate casual sexual encounters (Duguay, 2018).

The women I spoke with highlighted how Tinder's importing of Facebook data rarely provided sufficient information to instill confidence when swiping on others. While logging in through Facebook is no longer mandatory, integrating cross-platform self-representations remains the norm, as Tinder has added this functionality for Instagram and Spotify. Contrary to bootstrapping trust, Tinder's design is complicit with user deception by giving a false sense of verification when the information accrued does nothing to indicate user intentions for meeting others on the app. Through the minimal information cues in the swipe screen and Tinder's reliance on automation and sorting algorithms, its lack of human checkpoints leaves the work of discerning trustworthiness up to its users.

One of my side projects when researching Tinder involved looking at how people were using the app for anything but dating (Duguay, 2020). I amassed examples of profiles peddling goods and services, announcing gigs, and boosting political messages, but my favorite among these were the joke accounts. In 2014, journalist Joe Veix created a Tinder account as a dog named Hero and chronicled people's strange responses to his barrage of "Bark! Bark! Bark!" in message threads (Veix, 2014). Proving that on Tinder no one knows you're *not* a dog, these joke profiles provide evidence that setting up a fake account is not only possible but common. Given that the queer women I interviewed were largely using the app to pursue sexual and romantic relationships with other women, configuring their browsing settings to reflect this, they interpreted users with other intentions or qualities to be deceptive when they were filtered into browse mode despite these settings. Within this definition of deception, these women noted varying degrees of deceptive misrepresentation pertaining to users' qualities and intentions, ranging from entirely fake accounts— that is, accounts created by someone not represented in the profile—to the omission of pivotal pieces of information. These deceptive encounters often involved a few common perpetrators: heterosexual women, couples looking for threesomes, and men.

Since Tinder lacks a profile field for sexual identity, this personal information is challenging to discern. In my experience of swiping through profiles, I often wondered if Tinder was showing me every woman on the app, regardless of her settings, to make it seem like my odds of finding a match were better than they actually were. Like my interview participants, I developed a keen eye for spotting heterosexual women based on what Danaë, a nineteen-year-old student who is lesbian, coined the "straight-girl look." For her, this look was fraught with "duck face selfies" and other tropes of hyperfemininity. She was annoyed with the prevalence of heterosexual women who were "just looking for friends," to whom she wanted to say, "That's not what you use Tinder for—get friends in real life!" Similarly, Briana, who is also a student but is later in her twenties and queer, wished that there was a profile field for sexual identity so she could "know if that person is going to swipe on me or whether they're just looking for—like, if they're straight and looking for friends." Other dating apps contain such fields. OkCupid even has a functionality that hides the profiles of gay or bisexual-identified users from straight ones (OkCupid, 2019), effectively making it difficult for heterosexual people to clog up queer people's inboxes looking for their new gay best friend.

Phyllis, the law student in her early twenties whose profile opened chapter 1, explained that heterosexual women's profiles often contained faux performances of nonheterosexuality: "They're hanging off the arms of dudes or if they've got pictures of themselves almost kissing girls, like, they're *this* far apart and they're like, 'Oh my God, look at how gay I am!' and I'm like, 'No, that's like the straightest photo you could take.'" With the permeation of feminized lesbian chic imagery in the media in the 1990s and 2000s and the continued fetishization of lesbians through heterosexual pornography (Diamond, 2005; Jenefsky & Miller, 1998), such performances can be read as appealing to popular culture and heterosexual desirability. Danaë described the unspoken intention behind the straight-girl look: "I'm just on Tinder for friends/sleep with me and my boyfriend." She viewed these users as attempting to enhance their attractiveness to men through flirtation and allusions to sexual activity with other women.

While Tinder's one-on-one matching defaults toward monogamous relationship styles, two or more people can use one account to represent themselves. Most participants did not take issue with couples who were open about searching for nonmonogamous arrangements. Caitlin, a nurse in her midtwenties, noted that some couples stated in their profiles something along the lines of, "We're looking for someone to have fun with," and if that was not your thing, they were easy to "just screen out." But it was common for accounts to only display pictures of one person in a heterosexual relationship, generally the female given that they were trying to appeal to women seeking women, and then reveal their intention upon matching. This occupation of time and attention frustrated Julia, an accountant in her late twenties who is gay: "Some of them you can't tell from the profile. It might just be photos of the girl and not a girl and a guy." She observed that some users even claimed to be single in their profiles, only to reveal later that this was not the case. Although fewer and fewer people list their relationship status on Facebook (Robards & Lincoln, 2016), it is surprising that Tinder does not attempt to import this information. Participants spoke of unexpectedly encountering only heterosexual couples and not same-gender couples, reflecting the fetishization of rare "unicorn" bisexual women willing to have sex with heterosexual couples. With the majority of interviewees noticing couples while swiping (not just bisexual or pansexual individuals), heterosexual couples' persistence in pursuing women whose sexual identities excluded attraction to men also perpetuates discourses that question or deny the possibility of female sexuality without men, thus heterosexualizing lesbian identities (Jackson & Gilbertson, 2009).

Even women who specified they only wanted to be shown women came across accounts seemingly operated by men. At the minor end of deception, several clearly male-presenting profiles surfaced in their browse screens. Participants were divided over whether this was a glitch in Tinder's sorting algorithm or these individuals had manually switched their gender, which was automatically imported from Facebook but could be changed in the settings screen. Some women conjectured that perhaps these men aimed to sway their desires by appearing in their searches. More severe cases of deception involved what Julia referred to as catfishing accounts. A term popularized by the docudrama *Catfish* (2010) and subsequent reality show (2012–) of the same name, to *catfish* is to create a fake identity for the purpose of luring a person into a relationship. Julia recounted, "There was this one [account] that was a girl and then they're like, 'Can you send me some photos? Send it to this number.' And then I got my housemate to call the number and it was a guy's voicemail." After similar scenarios happened several times, she developed heuristics for identifying deceptive accounts, looking to see whether they had a lack of Facebook friends or a fairly empty Instagram account. She asserted, "If they start talking dirty straightaway or they ask for nudes, then it's a guy."

While there is not always a clear way to tell that such accounts are run by men, multiple studies document the rampant male-instigated aggressive sexual solicitations, harassment, and threats of violence that women experience on dating websites and apps (Gillett, 2018; Hess & Flores, 2018; Shaw, 2016). This demonstrates that app designers' concerns are misplaced in ensuring people are "real," since better checks and reporting systems are needed when real people treat others in sexually exploitative, threatening, and dehumanizing ways. The bisexual and pansexual women I interviewed aired major concerns about trying to meet men through Tinder. ThunderGoddess, a consultant in her midthirties who picked a creative pseudonym during our interview, felt that men treated her like "a walking vagina" in their aggressive sexual pickup lines. Similarly, Caitlin decided not to bother with dating men through Tinder due to her past experiences with sexually aggressive matches. She kept this in mind when initiating conversations with women: "I'm very, very careful not to be too aggressive, reflecting on my own experiences, particularly with men." While deception can be frustrating and time-consuming when matching with others whose intentions, relationships, or qualities are not compatible with one's own, Tinder use becomes dangerous when it facilitates interactions with aggressive and coercive individuals.

These women's experiences reflect a broader sexualized and misogynist culture of use stemming from Tinder's imagined affordances. Recalling Nagy and Neff's (2015) argument that a technology's users, materiality, and designer intentions shape its imagined affordances, it follows that expectations about how Tinder should be used arise from this combination. Material qualities of the swipe as rapid, binary, and visually oriented combine with designer intentions revealed in Tinder's early marketing campaigns. The app was first promoted to American fraternities and sororities (Marinova, 2016), which run rampant with sexual double standards that socially reward men for pursuing sex, positioning women as sexual gatekeepers and often punishing them reputationally if they do participate in casual sex (Bogle, 2008; DeSantis, 2007). Early Tinder launch parties also took place in nightclubs, with now-removed YouTube showreels juxtaposing the app's use with clips featuring female models and alcohol consumption. Through both approaches to popularizing the app, Tinder became associated with youth, nightlife, and, most pronouncedly, casual sexual encounters. Popular media reinforced this association among users through op-eds, late-night comedy bits, memes, and entertainment news. Among the most memorable of these is a *Vanity Fair* piece by Nancy Jo Sales (2015), "Tinder and the Dawn of the 'Dating Apocalypse,'" which paints a dystopian picture of a world in which millennials are no longer capable of romance thanks to Tinder relegating them to noncommittal hook-ups.

The imagined affordances of Tinder for hooking up and gender-based scripts associated with heterosexual casual sex contribute to women's experiences of sexual aggression when using the app. These experiences are evidenced through the Instagram account @tindernightmares, where women anonymously submit screenshots of Tinder exchanges that reflect "toxic masculine performances" attempting to exert a patriarchal hierarchy by sending hypersexual and objectifying messages (Hess & Flores, 2018). Several women I spoke with were reluctant to report sexually aggressive behavior on Tinder due to its prevalence and normalization. Caitlin told me, "I'm kind of sure that it's perfectly appropriate to some people." Jean Burgess, Nicholas Suzor, and I (Duguay et al., 2018) posit that this dominant culture of use combines with weak prohibitions in Tinder's terms of service against "misleading" conduct and the app's minimal features for taking action to reinforce women's feelings of having little recourse.

These intrusions and other qualities of the app made partner seeking difficult for queer women. From frequent "Tinder tourists" seeking a quick hook-up during a vacation to participants' sense that Tinder's geolocational information was not reliable enough to put them in contact with others at a nightclub, several participants recalled regularly and rapidly swiping through all of the women near them. Laura, a project manager in her midthirties who is pansexual, noted that this was specifically a problem for women seeking women: "My friend and I would just sit beside each other on a quiet Sunday night and be like, 'Let's play Tinder together.' . . . She was interested in men only, and at the time, I was women only, and I'd be done in ten minutes and she could go on, and on, and on."

Frequent encounters with deceptive users and the ability to quickly swipe through all nearby female profiles indicated a woeful scarcity of other queer women. However, Tinder still seemed to present the best prospects for dating. Other women-specific apps were often discontinued because they lacked the volume of users needed to keep them afloat. ThunderGoddess observed: "The concept of, like, a Crushr or Vagster or whatever they have for queer women, I think that it's a good idea that works in London, San Francisco, you know, LA and New York, but if you're outside of a place like that, there just isn't the critical mass to be able to make it work." Tinder's embeddedness in heterosexual culture was simultaneously the reason that queer women had to deal with heterosexual women attempting to capitalize on faux lesbian desirability, heterosexual couples looking for a third, and toxic masculinity, as well as the reason for the app's widespread uptake and financial sustainability. Given this, the women I spoke with found ways to make Tinder work for them by increasing the salience of their sexual identity with the intention of dissuading deceptive users and attracting other queer women.

SALIENCE THROUGH RECOGNIZABILITY

Laura proclaimed that she was not worried about whether other women on Tinder could tell that she identified as pansexual. She shrugged as she said, "If other women have 'women' as their interest, then that's how they're going to see me and that's how they're going to know I'm interested in women." However, her profile photos demonstrated that she had not merely left this up to the app's settings. They showed an array of short and brightly colored hairstyles, ending on a particularly gripping image of Laura blowing smoke rings, her face decorated with David Bowie–like paint interspersed with iridescent gems, accentuated by a silver-frosted, androgynous hairstyle. While her appearance did not communicate a particular sexual identity, it certainly transgressed normative expressions of feminine and heterosexual desirability in very salient ways.

The women I spoke with used profile photos, biographies, and media references to increase the salience of their sexual identity within the constraints of Tinder's profile design and functionalities. Indications of sexual identity worked most effectively when they were recognizable, either as deviations from heteronormativity, as was the case with Laura's photos, or in association with well-known lesbian or other LGBTQ stereotypes, tropes, and cultural trappings. For some participants, photos were a seamless way to communicate sexual identity. Bec, who is in her early thirties and between jobs, identifies interchangeably as gay or lesbian and felt that this should be clear from her tomboy style: "I don't feel the need to tell everyone necessarily, like flat out . . . people should be able to pick up on that. In my real life, I present pretty much as gay, you can tell [by] looking at me, basically." Other women included photos of themselves at Pride festivals, wearing rainbow accessories or plaid clothing, or engaging in sports.

However, photos were not always salient enough, according to some interviewees, especially those who did not feel their visual self-representation indicated their sexual identity. Danaë noted that her photos did not scream "She's gay!" and progressively added details to the short bio (biography) field of her profile. "So, I just did the two-girl emoticon, which I kept seeing on other people's profiles. . . . But then it always really annoyed me when people didn't have anything written." With a five-hundred-character limit, Tinder's constraint on user self-descriptions encourages minimal detail and fosters a platform vernacular of bios containing only a couple of emoji or no writing at all. Danaë's frustration with the confusion this bred led her to retain the 👭 emoji but also list "I love theatre, festivals, markets, films, books, and traveling. Oh, and girls 😘," with the final remark making her attraction to women explicit.

Gertie, a midthirties accountant who is gay, added the two-women-holding-hands emoji shortly after creating her account: "I realized that's what everyone was doing, so I did it just to help out, I guess." With the predominance of Apple's rendition of the Unicode character, this standardized representation of white women (or yellow, Apple's standard skin tone, with other options only added in later years) in feminine clothing became a recognizable symbol of female, same-gender attraction on Tinder. The Apple emoji format was so common that Phyllis panicked when it looked different on her Android phone: "I was almost going to return [the phone] when I got it, because I'm like, 'That is totally not obvious enough. I can't see it.'" This specific emoji served as digital shorthand for queer women's sexual identity, becoming popular within Tinder's cultures of use despite its lack of diversity and the traditional gender expression it perpetuates.

Like Danaë, other participants felt that written statements about sexual identity were the clearest way to communicate this information. Julia's bio declared "100% gay" as a deterrent to heterosexual couples searching for threesomes. In contrast, Caitlin's bio sacrificed accuracy for recognizability. She wrote "bi," short for bisexual, instead of "homoflexible" or "pansexual," which are the identifiers she feels most comfortable using to represent her attraction to people across a gender spectrum. She explained, "If you said 'pan,' it may require further explanation, depending on who you're talking to. If you said 'homoflexible,' again, further explanation, so it's a convenience thing." Despite an increasing number of celebrities and media personalities identifying as pansexual in the 2010s, such as Miley Cyrus's highly publicized coming out (Setoodeh, 2016), Caitlin still felt that "bisexual" was the most recognizable descriptor related to her sexual identity.

Those who referred to LGBTQ media or personalities assumed that the lifestyles associated with particular sexual identities would lead one to accrue such cultural knowledge. Phyllis quizzed her matches by asking, "Oh, do you watch *Orange Is the New Black*? Or, have you seen *The Rocky Horror Picture Show* before?" As mentioned in chapter 1, *Orange Is the New Black* (2013–19) was popular across audience demographics but particularly known for its LGBTQ characters and storylines, while *The Rocky Horror Picture Show* (1975) has become a queer cult classic. Phyllis felt that this kind of questioning could help her to pinpoint another's sexual identity, based on how that person interpreted particular media representations. She shared one elaborate strategy: "A really good question that used to work is, if you ask them if they thought Kristen Stewart was gay. And if they said yes, then they're gay because a straight girl would not know anything about Kristen Stewart being gay." This made sense during our interview, since the celebrity who starred as Bella in the iconic heterosexual teenage drama *Twilight* (2008) had not yet made her 2017 debut on *Saturday Night Live* declaring that she was "so gay" to the show's millions of viewers (Michelson, 2017). Tabloids had merely circulated hypotheses about Stewart's sexuality up to that point. "But," Phyllis continued with her hypothesis, "if they said [she's] bisexual, then they're bisexual because only a bisexual would say that Kristen Stewart's bisexual because she's sleeping with dudes and chicks." I let this sink in for a moment. Although paparazzi had brought much attention to Stewart's relationships with women, their reports often desexualized and heterosexualized these interactions. For example, the *Daily Mail* (2015) described Alicia Cargile as Stewart's "live-in gal pal," a term reflective of the media's frequent erasure of lesbian and bisexual women (McBean, 2016). According to Phyllis's logic, bisexual women would claim Stewart as representing bisexuality, especially in efforts to counteract widespread bi-erasure, which lesbians may actually reinforce by claiming Stewart as one of their own despite her relationships with men. These responses to such a seemingly simple question belied personal biases and associations that Phyllis read as supporting matches' claims to particular sexual identities.

Representing sexual identity in accordance with what others understand to be recognizable and reliable can be challenging. Beyond being media savvy, someone responding to Phyllis's question must also have a grasp of how certain celebrities are received within a broader context of LGBTQ media commentary. The previous examples also exhibit a skillful capacity to meld stereotypical and traditional indicators of nonheterosexuality with digital formats, yielding photos, emoji, and concise bios that communicate sexual identity. These ways of modulating salience reflect emergent forms of digital literacy comprised of more than an understanding of *how to* use Tinder. This digital literacy fuses references to LGBTQ culture with digital practices in ways that these individuals imagine will resonate with other queer women. Design researcher Lindsay Ferris and I have called this Tinder's "lesbian digital imaginary" (Ferris & Duguay, 2019), building on the concept of imagined affordances (Nagy & Neff, 2015) to identify that which emerges from collective imaginings of identity made tangible through app affordances. We theorize that a digital imaginary is constituted by this fusion of cultural and digital signaling practices meant to be recognized by an imagined community of people who are thought to be similar to each other. This concept extends theories of one's "imagined audience" on social media (Marwick & boyd, 2011; Litt, 2012), mentioned in chapter 1, to identify how individuals approach such an unknowable audience based on imagined similarities. Many indicators of sexual identity that my participants (as well as the women in Ferris's research) chose to accentuate specifically spoke to recognizable stereotypes associated with lesbian identities. As these indicators were repeated and became common across Tinder among women seeking women, they gave rise to a lesbian digital imaginary as a suite of signals that stands in for a range of female nonheterosexual identifications. These signals of combined cultural and digital literacy provided a user-constructed filter for identifying and dismissing heterosexual women, men, and couples in browse mode.

However, a default toward indicators of lesbian identity reflects existing biases and exclusions among LGBTQ people, which also play out on Tinder. The valorization of normative femininity among queer women is frequently reflected in who garners the most attention on dating websites and apps (Hightower, 2015). Several of the women I spoke with acknowledged this hierarchy, with Danaë describing a ranking system for her dating preferences: "So, my level of femininity or a little bit higher, but I can also go down to the chapstick area too. But yeah, I just personally don't find the butch look attractive." She identifies "Chapstick" as a category of slightly less feminine queer women in an unspoken juxtaposition to "lipstick lesbians," who are stereotypically conceived to be extremely feminine in their fashion and activities. The *Urban Dictionary*'s top example of how to use the term *lipstick lesbian* illustrates a dismissal of more masculine, or "butch," women as undesirable: "If I wanted to date someone who looked like a man, I'd find a man. Where are all the lipstick lesbians?" (Lyric, 2004).

Participants were tongue in cheek about this gender bias and their focus on homonormative standards of attractiveness, favoring slender women with higher-paying jobs, with one interviewee admitting that this reflected "a little bit of snobbery." Their preferences are undoubtedly shaped by broader structures that reinforce perceptions of desirability, which sociologist Emerich Daroya (2018) discusses as hierarchies of erotic capital. Daroya observes these hierarchies among men on Grindr, where they reinforce conventional masculine expression, normative body types, and whiteness as pinnacles of desirability. Although the women I interviewed did not mention race specifically, the pale figures of the "two women holding hands" emoji and frequent references to white celebrities as litmus tests for sexual identity similarly contribute to racial hierarchies. The use of such indicators is reinforced through racial biases in technological design, contributing to the default whiteness of emoji, which has been slow to change due to developers' color-blind racism, reflected in assertions of the neutrality of technical design choices (Miltner, 2020). Similarly, Tinder's design choices to emphasize visual displays and include occupation and education as some of the only default profile fields play a role in shaping how users filter each other according to normative standards of attractiveness and socioeconomic status.

Tinder's lesbian digital imaginary can also be seen as reinforcing existing boundaries of exclusion and creating new ones in relation to sexual and gender identity. Psychology researchers Tara Pond and Panteá Farvid (2017) found that bisexual women on Tinder self-represent using indicators of lesbian identity to avoid enduring biphobia. This resonates with the women in my research who identified as bisexual or pansexual but sought to indicate nonheterosexuality visually rather than by using a specific identity label that would exclude them from the searches of those looking for lesbians. Further, the association of lesbian identity with cisgender female identity combines with Tinder's binary gender categories to erase gender-nonbinary, genderfluid, and transgender users. In response to user outcry over the mass reporting and blocking of transgender individuals, Tinder eventually added a profile field in 2017 allowing individuals to select from a range of gender identities beyond male and female (O'Brien, 2017). However, browse settings still force users to choose from seeking men or women (or both), with no way to specifically seek transgender users or for transgender individuals to filter out transphobic users. Laura remarked on this difficulty: "If I'm pansexual and I'm interested in meeting a trans person, that's not an option for me, so it is limiting in that aspect." Although transgender users can now specify their gender identity on their profiles, they may be dissuaded by continued blocking and hostility (Riotta, 2019).

Last, the level of both LGBTQ cultural literacy and digital literacy required to signal oneself as part of the lesbian digital imaginary may exclude some users who are indeed queer women but fail to give off the *right* signals. What if someone has no clue who Kristen Stewart is? What if this person does not know what to include in photos or is oblivious about emoji? This demand for a certain level of literacy pertaining to digital and LGBTQ cultures assumes that individuals are adept in both, which may not be the case for people who are just coming out, those who are unfamiliar with dating apps, or other subsets of Tinder users.

Despite these complications, the women I interviewed found ways to negotiate Tinder's affordances and cultures of use to create profiles they felt represented their sexual identities. For some women who identified as lesbian or gay, signaling this through stereotypes was useful and could be done in humorous or ironic ways. Others, whose sexual identities did not fit these highly recognizable categories, found creative ways to signal nonheterosexuality and even poke fun at or disrupt clean-cut categories. This could be achieved through more fluid, edgy, and queer self-representations, such as Laura's shimmering Bowie makeup alongside her disregard for identity labels.

RECALIBRATING FOR INCREASED SALIENCE

Heightening the salience of information about sexual identity calls for the modulation of personal identifiability and reach. Many women I interviewed were concerned about balancing these dynamics on two levels: first, to maintain their Tinder profile within the app's specific social context, and second, to preserve their safety when matching with and meeting new people. The first concern arose from their profiles' conveying sexual identities and desires within the framing of Tinder's reputation as a hook-up app and associated negative sexual scripts (Albury, 2018), as well as the enduring stigmatization of hook-up and dating apps more broadly (Leong, 2016). Participants took concerted measures to ensure that despite Tinder's importing of Facebook data, their self-representations on the app did not reach back to their Facebook audiences. Since at this time only Facebook photos could be uploaded to Tinder, several women created specific Facebook photo albums for this purpose, using different images for dating than for everyday self-representation.

When Julia contemplated using Tinder for the first time, she was worried that the app would inadvertently out her to her Facebook contacts. Having recently broken up with her male fiancé, she was not ready to tell people she was dating women, so she created another Facebook account: "I had a gay one and a straight one. . . . I'd add people that I talked to [on Tinder] on Facebook and I didn't want everyone else to see that, so I kept it separate." Separating audiences across different accounts or platforms is a common way to manage reach, with people increasingly creating secondary accounts. In the years since this interview, creating Finstas—"fake" Instagram accounts—has become a popular way for individuals to maintain an intimate and less-curated self-representation with smaller audiences, separated from their "real" or more followed public accounts (Xiao et al., 2020). However, while Instagram has introduced features to make account switching easy, Facebook retains an emphasis on holding only one account as a reflection of a singular, authentic identity. As such, Julia would have had to work to create and maintain two separate accounts. While she eventually merged the accounts as she came out to more people, containing the reach of information about her sexual identity was necessary at such a transitional time in her life.

Tinder's design contravenes this desire to maintain a separation between Facebook contacts and potential dates. When browsing profiles, the app displays users' mutual friends, presumably as an indicator of compatibility. Instead, Danaë interpreted this as a red flag: "It's kind of creepy when you come across complete strangers and they have so many mutual friends, and you're like, 'How don't I know about you? Why has no one told me about you?'" She assumed that her friends would have already introduced her to any viable dates within her existing networks. Encountering friends through the app also called for a particular demeanor, which Laura termed "friendship etiquette," given that these friendships were established in other contexts but were now subject to Tinder's sexual framing. ThunderGoddess described a protocol through which she matched with existing contacts to be friendly but limited conversation: "We both acknowledge each other's presence, read each other's profile, make a comment about somebody else's profile . . . and then we go back to being stock standard friends." Notably, she and her friends do not comment on each other's profiles but only discuss mutual contacts. This approach shares similarities with what Goffman (1966) called "civil inattention," the practice of noticing but not paying concerted attention to others as they go about their business: the nod and smile as you pass someone on the sidewalk. The mobile dating version of civil inattention includes matching to say hi but avoiding discussion of, or focus on, personal disclosures in Tinder profiles intended for potential dates but not existing friends.

With Tinder's mobile use and geolocational functionality, individuals also managed their personal identifiability and the reach of their information in relation to their physical location. HotChocolate, another interviewee with a creative pseudonym who is in her midthirties, found it convenient to use Tinder during lulls at work, but she was also concerned about being outed to her homophobic co-workers. She noted, "I didn't feel that it was necessary to openly out myself at work because I'm there to work as a secretary. I'm not a lesbian secretary, I'm just a secretary" and kept her Tinder use from view. While the salience of sexual identity was useful for matching with previously unknown queer women, it also became a liability, since participants could not know when their profiles were being shown to people near them. Caitlin was prepared to delete her profile upon relocating for work: "There's no privacy when you're using social media in a small town." She did not want her Tinder profile to affect first impressions with new neighbors and colleagues. While co-situation on the app and in physical space can help queer women find each other, it can also backfire when individuals do not want to be recognizable on the app to proximate others.

In terms of preserving safety, participants' second level of concern, identity modulation involved adjusting personal identifiability and assessing others' identifiable information, often in ways that circumvented or supplemented Tinder's integration of Facebook data. Briana deleted the education and job information from her profile: "I think it's interesting to know somebody's occupation as a general sense, but to know if they're in a company—a small company—that might be problematic." Participants often omitted information from their profiles that could lead to the discovery of home or work addresses and other social media accounts. They also took measures to verify matches' personal information by layering multiple modes of communication and accessing several information sources. Bec followed two steps: "If you [look on] Facebook and then, at least, you speak to them on the phone, you get a good grasp of whether they're crazy or not." Other participants spoke of texting, looking at Instagram or Snapchat profiles, googling matches, and sending lengthy messages for days before meeting up. Information studies scholar Caroline Haythornthwaite's (2005) foundational concept of media multiplexity describes how people employ more forms of communication as their social bonds become stronger. This practice was also evident in the work of digital media scholar Elija Cassidy (2018), who observed that gay men often initiated contact on Gaydar, a gay social network, and then moved conversations to MSN Messenger or Facebook to get to know each other.

In Tinder's case, it is noteworthy that the app's integration of Facebook data did not forestall these practices of media multiplexity. Although Tinder imported highly personally identifiable information, accessing a match's Facebook account directly (by friending), communicating through one-on-one channels, and corresponding for longer durations gave participants the sense that this information was reliable as an accumulation of identity-related cues over time and through the revelation of intimate details. These layered interactions conveyed personal information that might not be readily available through Facebook and, by extension, Tinder profiles. Only after exchanging messages for days did Danaë feel confident enough in a match's trustworthiness to arrange a meetup at her house for "TV and cuddles," a version of "Netflix and chill" with less sexual expectation.[1] These steps set the foundation for a relationship that she was absolutely swooning over by the time we met for an interview. In other words, these multiple forms of exchange enabled matches to build intimacy with each other prior to meeting in person—something that was difficult to accomplish through Tinder's default focus on personally identifiable but sexually vacant information.

CONCLUSION: RECLAIMING IDENTITIES, BUILDING TRUST

This chapter has provided a look at the multifaceted processes of identity modulation in relation to Tinder and queer women's self-representation. Tinder's functionality for importing Facebook data and prepopulating user profiles illustrates how influential a platform can be in processes of identity modulation. To fully grasp Tinder's role in these processes, I find it useful to combine concepts across disciplines. Taking an actor network theory (ANT) perspective, it is possible to identify platforms and their features as nonhuman objects: they are indeed programmed by people, but the resulting app on a smartphone is nonetheless an object. Bruno Latour (1992), a focal philosopher of ANT, asserts that we often ask a lot of objects, since we delegate tasks to them that were once up to humans. He gives the example of a door that closes itself rather than requiring humans to do it; such objects with programmed step-by-step procedures are often perceived to be more reliable than humans. With the bootstrapping logic behind Tinder and related apps that automatically pull data from another source to compile an individual's presence, the tasks of identity building and self-representation become delegated to the platform.[2] These previously user-centered activities have given way to the automated production of platform-generated identities.

Through this delegation of self-representation, personal information from one context is placed into another. When objects are influential in shaping relationships within networks of people and things, Latour (2005) calls them "mediators," which "transform, translate, distort, and modify the meaning or the elements they are supposed to carry" (p. 39). Tinder and its functionality for Facebook integration are mediators in multiple ways: they alter how the imported data are displayed—feeding them into a visually heavy, swipe-able profile layout—and they show this information to new and different audiences. Through Tinder's geolocational features and mobile use, digital profiles also become anchored to physical locations. This poses complications for users with regard to managing self-representations, which must be approached differently from the in-person situations Goffman (1959) observed as well as from the electronic communications that Meyrowitz (1985) identified as disembedded from geography. Instead, as the women featured throughout the chapter showed, Tinder placed them in situations of "mobile intimacy" (Hjorth & Lim, 2012) in which the overlay of their physical and digital self-representations required management through the modulation of reach and personal identifiability.

However, Tinder is not merely an object, and this is where other perspectives are necessary for understanding its full impact on identity modulation. First, Tinder is a company, connected to a "platform ecosystem" (van Dijck et al., 2018) of other commercially owned digital properties. Facebook prompts users to exchange as much potentially profitable data as possible, eventually fostering a large enough pool of information for Tinder to rely on as a supposed form of user verification. Second, Tinder's business motives shape its role as an authority over users' conduct. The app's developers craft policies and make choices about what to allow and disallow. These policies tend to facilitate a lucrative male-dominant and heteronormative user base by having minimal repercussions for sexually aggressive behavior and by removing transgender people's accounts when they are flagged by transphobic users. Finally, Tinder has become a common tool in intimate life (Newett et al., 2017), to which the media and everyday users attach meaning. The app's early marketing, media coverage, and social media discussions[3] situate it within heteronormative and gender-normative dating scripts. With these different elements considered, Tinder can be understood not only as a technological object but also as emerging from social, cultural, and economic arrangements.

These arrangements provide the basis for Tinder's identity modulation dynamics, set out at the beginning of this chapter: importing information from Facebook provides a high level of personal identifiability; location-based features place moderate constraints upon reach; and a lack of profile fields for intimate information and the app's assumed role in facilitating heterosexual casual sex contribute to the reduced salience of other sexual identities. As such, queer women find themselves having to discern the intentions of others, as they are subject to varying degrees of deception from users who wish to engage with them in unwanted interactions. In response, the women I interviewed resisted their default platform-generated identities: they increased the salience of indicators of sexual identity in their profiles, often by drawing on recognizable symbols, stereotypes, or media, in ways that allowed them to claim part in a lesbian digital imaginary that both facilitated partner seeking and recreated hierarchies of desirability. They also recalibrated other dynamics of identity modulation, removing automatically imported information and making choices about *where* to use the app to temper personal identifiability and reach.

Although Tinder imports personally identifiable data from Facebook, it does not actually succeed in bootstrapping trust. Instead, individuals' identity modulation practices discussed in this chapter served to foster a sense of trustworthiness among queer women on the app. Their responses to Tinder's prepopulated profiles imbued their self-representations with more intimate personal information about sexual identity, often alongside indications of their desires, preferences, and relationship status. This kind of intimate information can establish common ground with others, as we will see further in subsequent chapters, and aligns intentions for matching—indicating what one is seeking and enabling an assessment of whether a potential date meets those criteria and is seeking the same. These women's identity modulation strategies also aimed to contain app-specific self-representations within Tinder while negotiating the gradual addition of other means of communication. These supplemental and resistant forms of identity modulation in response to Tinder's default arrangements were integral to really generating trust between users, which stemmed from consistent and intimate self-representations that could not be convincingly platform generated. As a result, these women shared with me stories about dates that led to friendship and romance as well as to relationships that lasted for years. Similarly, my date's willingness to text, add me as a Facebook friend, and eventually open up about her personal life is surely what made a right swipe into a relationship.

CHAPTER 3

#Lesbehonest

Reach through Self-Branding

On a sunny day in the park, two boys' T-shirts caught my attention. One that read "Million dollar smile" got me thinking about how this is a literal quality that some people are able to cultivate. People who gain recognition for talents like singing or acting may eventually generate enough fame to make money simply by showing up and smiling, such as through celebrity appearances. However, this sequence seems reversed for those who make it big through social media. Someone who has become a social media star might have started out by smiling in a photo posted to Instagram, initiating a relationship with a specific audience that was maintained and expanded until a large following was generated and brands took notice. These two paths to fortune are often conflated. For example, in one analytics agency's "Instagram Rich List" of top-grossing accounts (Hopper, 2019), celebrities and social media influencers are interspersed when sorted by follower count. However, when ranked by profit generation, celebrities clutter the top of the list, while social media stars' advertising pay rates start high and plummet rapidly, to the point where some are flashing smiles for just a few hundred bucks. I thought to myself, in a world where social media are often intertwined not only with our social but also our economic activity, a million-dollar smile might be what these children will need to make a living when they are older.

The other boy's T-shirt depicted an amplifier alongside the words "volume control" in block letters. Maybe the boys' parents did not think twice about the T-shirt slogans, but their combination seemed apt to me. Identity

Personal but Not Private. Stefanie Duguay, Oxford University Press. © Oxford University Press 2022.
DOI: 10.1093/oso/9780190076184.003.0003

modulation can be thought of as a form of volume control: adjusting the loudness of the most personal aspects of identity in different situations. As I mentioned in chapter 1, drawing an analogy to sound modulation originally inspired the concept of identity modulation. Though identity modulation is less like a single volume control and more like a DJ mixer, as people use the preset controls—the default platform affordances—to adjust the multiple dynamics of identity modulation. As will become evident throughout this chapter, such *volume control* is essential to even coming close to having a million-dollar smile on social media.

"Lesbehonest" is another phrase that one can find on T-shirts (honestly, search Etsy) and across the internet. I noticed its prominence as a hashtag on queer women's social media posts in 2015 and have seen it endure over the years alongside others (e.g., #girlswholikegirls, #gaygirl, #lezzigram, #lesbianfunhouse, #lesbianlove, and variations in spelling like #lezbehonest or #lesbihonest). Although its origin is difficult to pin down, online searches point to the phrase's popularization through the movie *Pitch Perfect* (2012). One scene in this story of an eclectic and underdog female a cappella group competing to win the national collegiate title, which has been heavily remediated in fan GIFs, portrays the group's attempt to get to know each other by sharing secrets. When one character, Cynthia Rose, who has an asymmetrical haircut and loose-fitting clothes, gets up to share something that she says is "hard for me to admit," the character "Fat Amy," played by the rambunctious Australian actress Rebel Wilson, whispers, "We all know where this is going." More audibly, Amy says, "Lesbehonest" as a portmanteau of "lesbian" and "let's be honest," implying that Cynthia Rose should come out because they already know she is a lesbian. The joke lies in Cynthia Rose's confession being instead about her gambling problem. When she mentions, without hesitation or fanfare, that she started gambling after breaking up with her girlfriend, Amy responds, "Whomp, there it is!" Her misplaced focus on coming out invokes humor because the audience knows that while Cynthia Rose's sexual identity is relevant, it is not the big reveal that Amy makes it out to be.

I have seen #lesbehonest used across Instagram and, previously, Vine less as an invocation to come out, as Amy intended, but more as a tongue-in-cheek declaration of lesbian identity. For example, in its inclusion on Vines showcasing tattoos or Instagram photos of couples kissing, it functions as a reflexive declaration, "Yes, this is very lesbian." Rather than an essentialist assertion—indeed there is nothing inherently lesbian about tattoos—it serves to reclaim particular fashions and stereotypes. Instead of a somber "Let's be honest, you're a lesbian" coming from someone else, individuals use the hashtag for a salient celebration of their identity and its everyday facets.

Simultaneously, this salience of lesbian identity features in the service of self-branding on social media. The hashtag places a user's posts among similar others and circulates them to audiences searching for identity-affirming content, facilitating the accrual of new followers. The rampant commercialization of sexual identity also renders it into an intelligible brand—a particular flavor or a niche—within a social media landscape where one is often selling oneself as the product. Performance studies scholar Theresa Senft (2008) was among the first to notice the demand for self-branding online. Her ethnography of women who streamed their lives online in the early 2000s was the canary in the coal mine for identifying emerging digital practices giving rise to a widespread sense of the self as "microcelebrity" (Senft, 2008, 2013). While conventional celebrities garner fame through their accumulation of wealth and status, setting them apart from everyday people, microcelebrities focus on building relationships with their audiences. They do so by emphasizing their likeness to, or re-latability with, their followers. Senft (2013) observes that microcelebrity practices have become mainstream as a general "commitment to deploying and maintaining one's online identity as if it were a branded good, with the expectation that others do the same" (p. 346). A phrase like "Lesbehonest," signaling shared identification and relatable humor, might compel you to both buy the T-shirt and follow the Instagrammer who hashtags posts with it (and who might be advertising the T-shirt in the first place).

While scholars and digital literacy agendas alike highlight the increasing role of self-branding and digital skills in economic participation (Davies & Eynon, 2018; Hearn, 2010), platforms put a personal spin on this impera-tive in two particular ways. First, social media can evidence one's skills and accomplishments, serving as a continuously updating curriculum vitae. It is common for people to showcase their occupations on social media, from design, cooking, and creative jobs to less conventionally depicted work in trades and farming (Sergi & Bonneau, 2016). Demonstrating employability is not relegated to business networking platforms such as LinkedIn, but permeates across platforms. Foundational communications scholar Nancy Baym (2018) observes that "work and personal identities blur" (p. 18) as social media self-promotion becomes relational. Self-branding is no longer about having a shiny website. Instead, it entails interweaving per-sonal aspects of identity with financially lucrative skills and attributes to build relationships across audiences, from adoring followers to potential employers.

Second, while people display their everyday jobs on social media, being a social media personality is an occupation in itself. Popular media has latched onto a specific term for these laborers: "influencers," which anthropologist Crystal Abidin (2018) succinctly defines as "vocational, sustained, and highly branded social media stars" (p. 71). While influencers often have occupational specializations, such as cooking (e.g., Hannah Hart), singing (e.g., Troye Sivan), and makeup artistry (e.g., James Charles), their skill sets and labor are geared toward building personal brands that gain the attention of followers, advertisers, and broadcast media. The influencer industry has become increasingly professionalized through opportunities for sponsorships, crossovers to broadcast networks, and merchandising.

But there is a big gap between everyday people posting about their jobs and influencers signing deals with financial returns. Influencers' brand sponsorships lack a standardized pay rate, making their work precarious and setting the bar incredibly high for raking in enough cash to pay the bills. Even so, the influencer industry shapes how others view social media platforms and the possibilities they hold. Since the same platforms sustain everyday activity alongside influencers' ascent to fame, individuals sense that expending more effort toward self-branding could lead to economic and social gains. Influencers and broadcast media perpetuate this myth that *social media star* is an accessible occupation, obscuring existing wealth, social connections, and other behind-the-scenes factors leading to success (Duffy & Wissinger, 2017).

On the other side of this equation, platforms benefit from users' self-branding activity. Theorist Tiziana Terranova (2000) asserts that individuals' digital production constitutes "free labor" in the digital economy, which individuals may voluntarily enact for pleasurable outcomes, such as building communities, but is also exploited by corporations who rely on this activity to keep their digital properties fresh. Although writing before the social media boom, Terranova's argument is illustrative of social media's reliance on user-generated content for its value production: Facebook's stock would plummet if everyone stopped posting tomorrow because there would be nothing to attract users and no eyes for advertisements. Digital media is entrenched in what is often referred to as the "attention economy" (Goldhaber, 1997), where multiple actors vie for attention among volumes of online content. Media scholars Carolin Gerlitz and Anne Helmond (2013) add precision to these discussions by defining the "like economy" as that which emphasizes the economic value of the social, where "user interactions are instantly transformed into comparable forms of data and presented to other users in a way that generates more traffic and engagement" (p. 1349). While they focus on how social media infrastructures are configured to encourage, measure, and derive value from this engagement, users also respond to this economy. Research reveals that individuals expend concerted effort, conceptualized as labor, toward self-branding, networking, and relationship maintenance with the aim of fostering potentially profitable social media engagement (Abidin, 2018; Baym, 2018; Duffy, 2017; Marwick, 2016; Raun, 2018; Senft, 2008).

When identity modulation features in social media use for building capital—cultural, monetary, or both—it becomes part of individuals' labor. More succinctly, identity modulation in the service of self-branding constitutes labor. This chapter pivots toward a focus on two platforms where people have been known to work toward influencer status: Instagram and Vine in its heyday. Taking account of how these platforms' affordances are conducive to extending reach, especially through features for producing and circulating attention-grabbing media, I draw on ten interviews with queer women (eight Instagrammers, two Viners) conducted in 2016.[1] I also examine the content they posted alongside a broader analysis of posts with queer women's hashtags circulating in 2015–16. While photos and videos belied that queer women on these platforms clearly mobilized sexual identity as part of their self-branding, further investigation through interviews revealed their labor of identity modulation.

Through modulation of reach and salience, these women carried out three specific forms of labor to garner attention for their jobs, side gigs, and hobbies while bolstering engagement from followers. Their efforts involved intimate affective labor toward building relatability through personal disclosure, developmental aesthetic labor honing the skills required to portray such a persona, and aspiring relational labor reaching out to established celebrities and influencers to capture their attention and followings. Sexual identity featured across this labor in the revelation of intimate details, display of identity-related fashion, and as a common ground for relationship building. However, identity modulation was also necessary for these women's management of their extended reach, as they attempted to separate audiences across platforms, used pseudonyms to reduce personal identifiability, and modified the salience of sexual identity in relation to overlapping audiences. Examining identity modulation as a form of labor channeled into self-branding highlights a key tension in the monetization of personal disclosure: the creative sharing of oneself can simultaneously be experienced as empowerment and exploitation.

It is not by chance that Instagram and Vine have contributed to the rise of many influencers across niche and mainstream markets. Each platform presents affordances for attracting attention and drawing engagement from audiences. On Instagram, these affordances center on the app's distinctive introduction of image filters and the normative practices of aesthetic presentation associated with them. In contrast, Vine's 6.5-second looping video galvanized viewers' attention through action-packed audiovisual qualities. These key functionalities are flanked by features for engagement, such as hashtagging and "like" buttons, enabling the broad circulation of content. The following brief descriptions of each app provide background for this and the next chapter while also identifying how such affordances shape identity modulation by providing the possibility of a far reach for self-representations.

Instagram's "Frequently Asked Questions" section once asserted that the app was designed to remedy the problem of mediocre-looking mobile photos, a common plight of early smartphone cameras. Launched in 2010 by two Stanford University graduates, Kevin Systrom and Mike Krieger, Instagram, and specifically the app's photo filters, provided a solution for enhancing images' visual appeal. However, filters were not just technical presets for adjusting a digital photo's saturation, fade, or other qualities; they also presented a means to access and exhibit a "hipster" aesthetic that was on the rise in the 2010s. This aesthetic tempered individual expression with cultural knowledge of, and nostalgic affinity for, objects of the past, especially older technologies (Schiermer, 2014). Instagram's original icon resembling a 1970s Polaroid camera indicated an aspiration toward this aesthetic, alongside filter names like "1977" directly referencing past temporalities (Zappavigna, 2016). According to visual culture scholars Lisa Chandler and Debra Livingston (2016), this reintroduction of an analog aesthetic counteracts the capacity for digital technology to generate repetitive and mundane images. They highlight how filters intentionally reintroduce the flaws of analog film development processes (e.g., chemical spots) to give photos a sense of distinctiveness. Thus, Instagram filters provided users with the means to demonstrate individuality and the ability to (re) create a particular timely aesthetic, producing eye-catching images with the potential to spark engagement.

As the nostalgic hipster aesthetic waned in popularity, Instagram adjusted accordingly with new filters and a redesign in 2016, ditching the Polaroid icon for a multitonal, abstract camera (Leaver, Highfield, & Abidin, 2020). However, the discursive framing and practices associated with filters have set a high bar for images posted to the app. In its early years, the company blog showcased users who were stunning photographers, recommending them to new users as model accounts to follow. By 2015, when I first conducted the walkthrough method with the app, its description in Apple's App Store invoked users to "transform your everyday photos and videos into works of art." From everyday food shots to photos of war, the app's filters have been used expansively to beautify and render all subjects Instagrammable (Alper, 2014; Kohn, 2015).

With Facebook's acquisition of Instagram in 2012, ushering in app-embedded advertising, and celebrities rapidly joining the platform, users' works of art became intertwined with the presentation of commercial products and lifestyles as an aesthetic of glamour.[2] Communications scholar Alice Marwick (2015) observes a dominant "iconography of glamour, luxury, wealth, good looks, and connections" among Instagram's visual media. She argues that such content is indicative of individuals' aspirations to mimic celebrity styles to attract attention, generating "Instafame." While Marwick underscores that Instafamous practices reflect the permeation of celebrity culture and conspicuous consumption on Instagram, they also align with contemporary imperatives of self-branding. According to media scholar Sarah Banet-Weiser (2012), marketing in late capitalism has interwoven a ubiquitous brand culture with everyday activities and relationships. Within this brand culture, authenticity has become an important facet of self-branding—one that is no longer removed from the market but instead performed through practices of consumption. Therefore, using filters that enable the display of individuality and cultural agility to showcase oneself and one's goods in accordance with celebrity and brand culture communicates forms of authenticity and relatability conducive to building a following. Through these aesthetic tools and practices, Instagram facilitates a far reach for self-representations.[3]

Vine, on the other hand, offered few content editing tools but presented a different format for grabbing attention: short 6.5-second looping videos. Originally created by technology developers Dom Hofmann, Colin Kroll, and Rus Yusupov, Vine was reportedly acquired for US$30 million by Twitter, which officially launched the app in 2013 (Constine, 2016). Media coverage hailed it as "Instagram for video" (Peterson, 2013), since Instagram only added video functionality months after Vine's release and had yet to develop dedicated sections of the app for Stories or Reels. Yet Vine's developers shared a vision through the company blog that blended Twitter and Instagram. Blog entries first celebrated the app's release as "a new mobile service that lets you create and share beautiful, short looping videos" and later infused it with Twitter's mandate toward information exchange: "We want to make it easier for people to come together to share and discover what's happening in the world. . . . We also believe constraint inspires creativity, whether it's through a 140-character Tweet or a six second video."[4] Vine's blog showcased beautiful landscape footage and intricate stop-motion videos, encouraging the use of additional equipment and techniques to produce polished videos despite the app's simple tap-to-record functionality and time limit on videos. It also featured Vines by celebrities, attempting to foster a luxury appeal similar to Instagram's. In the first Vine ever posted, founder Dom Hofmann depicted a glamorous life moment, recording a French waiter preparing his order of steak tartare. However, unlike Instagram, Vine's absence of features supporting the production of a glamorized aesthetic led to creative user derivations that capitalized on the capture of raw footage. Hofmann's steak tartare video was about as far as one could get from the spontaneous, rapid-fire, and humor-filled Vines that would eventually populate the platform.

While the looping media format was not new, Vine couched it within a novel configuration of affordances. Social media users were already familiar with looping GIFs, which curator Jason Eppink (2014) defines as "an otherwise short, silent, looping untitled moving image" (p. 298). He notes that GIFs often encompass multiple images displayed in succession and circulate easily across platforms, generally without the start, pause, or stop buttons that accompany more formal video formats. Similarly, Vines circulated widely through seamless cross-platform posting and broke free from traditional video controls, which the developers denounced as giving "the impression that you're using a dusty video camera." Vines also combined the loop with sound and a fixed duration, providing affordances that media scholar Tim Highfield (2015) and I have observed users harnessing in three key ways: creating a narrative arc, with a single user often playing multiple roles while storytelling; generating affective intensity through first-person address paired with emotive speech or music; and packing a density of detail into videos with excitement culminating at the end. Captivating stories, affect, and detail all invited viewers to watch videos repeatedly as they looped automatically.

While the loop captivated viewers, its repetitive and simple format aligned with practices of online humor to establish Vines within meme culture. People participate in and share a meme when it is easy to replicate and provides a memorable hook for creative elaboration (Shifman, 2014). An iconic example from Vine's history is Diamonique Shuler's (@ Dom) video featuring a woman singing "do it for the Vine" to a young girl. Twice the girl responds "I ain't gonna do it," and the third time she breaks into dancing while the woman taps out a beat on the arm of her chair. The dialogue's repetition, along with the video's built-in loop, imbued this Vine with a rhythm that spurred others to like, share, and recreate it in different scenarios. While this video's huge reception cannot be directly connected to Vine's branding, the app eventually adopted "Do it for the Vine" as its tagline.[5]

Instagram's filtered aesthetics and Vine's loops are not the only affordances of these platforms that shape self-representations. However, they play a prominent role in technological arrangements that enhance individuals' reach in their processes of identity modulation through the attention they garner. A glamorous Instagram photo is often circulated to many eyes, while a humorous Vine video was known to spread quickly as users referenced the original to make their own derivatives. With the potential offered by these platforms for amplifying reach, users tailored their labor to direct attention toward their personal brand with hopes of garnering potentially lucrative engagement.

SELF-BRANDING WITH SEXUAL IDENTITY

On a Monday long past, lesbian burlesque dancer Queenie posted a #moonday photo to Instagram, participating in the hashtag trend of welcoming the week with a photo of one's butt—clothed or as naked as Instagram allows. The image displayed her with her partner, facing away from the camera to show matching rainbow underwear and cutie mark tattoos. Cutie marks are symbols on the haunches of characters from *My Little Pony*, a long-standing media franchise that has become enveloped in LGBTQ fandom. A white woman in her early thirties, Queenie sported Rainbow Dash's symbol, a rainbow lightning bolt, while her partner Emi, a biracial Asian and white genderqueer individual around the same age, displayed Soarin's golden lightning bolt with wings. The post's hashtags ensured it would turn up in searches relating to this fandom (e.g., #cutiemarktattoos, #rainbowdashcutiemark), butts (e.g., #assassassassass), and queer women (e.g., #lesbiansofinstagram, #dykesofinstagram, #tattooedlesbians). Additionally, Queenie included a unique "couple hashtag," #rainbowdashandsoarin4ever, as a declaration about their relationship that also made their photos easily searchable.

Queenie's #moonday post functioned as a form of personal self-representation while also contributing toward the self-brand she was building to promote her work as a burlesque dancer and model. Media studies scholar Alison Hearn (2010) observes that social media have given rise to a digital reputation economy, whereby individuals must expend labor "to direct human meaning-making and self-identity in highly motivated and profitable ways" (p. 423). The women I spoke with tended to represent their lives, families, and relationships on Instagram and Vine while aiming to garner fans, clients, and customers for their existing jobs and side gigs. On top of this, they kept in mind a (somewhat mythical) possibility of monetizing their social media activity through influencer-like approaches.

Communications scholar Brooke Duffy (2017) refers to such hopeful efforts toward success in digital economies as "aspirational labor," involving performances of authenticity, the formation of instrumental relationships, and entrepreneurial alignment of one's self-brand with commercial brands and commodity goods. In previous analysis (Duguay, 2019), I have proposed that aspirational labor forms a stepping stone to moving into a more consistent approach of what Nancy Baym (2018) calls "relational labor," constituted by "the ongoing, interactive, affective, material, and cognitive work of communicating with people over time to create structures that can support continued work" (p. 19). While Baym mainly observes the relational labor involved in being a musician, as music promotion has largely migrated to platforms, she notes that relational labor is increasingly key to the success of workers across individualized, entrepreneurial gig work.

There are, however, growing pains involved in aspiring to make it big or trying to look like you already have. Many of the women I interviewed were in this striving stage of self-promotion, teaching themselves the skills and techniques necessary to harness Instagram's and Vine's reach for their social and economic aims. Existing literature on microcelebrity insightfully reveals multiple modes of labor that are often obscured or rendered invisible in influencers' performances of having fun or doing what they love (Abidin, 2016; Duffy, 2017). The queer women I spoke with brought to light how these modes of labor look when they are conducted within this aspirational stage and involve identity modulation to integrate sexual identity into self-brands. Such a combination gives rise to what I have termed (1) *intimate affective labor* of sharing intimate personal details through relatable self-disclosure; (2) *developmental aesthetic labor* of acquiring and practicing skills to execute a specific appearance or persona that resonates with target audiences, which are often identity based; and (3) *aspiring relational labor* of attempting to build relationships with established social media influencers and celebrities based on a common ground of shared identity. Across these modes of labor, interviewees drew on platform affordances to elevate their reach while modulating the salience of their sexual identity, emphasizing it to foster intimacy, tailoring its expression into a recognizable brand, and highlighting it as the rationale for relationship building.

Disclosure and displays of sexual identity, as well as lives and relationships shaped by sexual identity, featured in queer women's Instagram photos and Vine videos to convey intimacy and foster affect. Take, for example, posts by Chrissy, an African American woman in her midtwenties who works a day job as a teacher's aide while promoting her crafts and paintings for sale through social media. Interspersed with posts showing her latest artwork, she often depicted humorous scenes involving her wife. One Vine clip captioned, "When your babe gives you the stink face cuz you tryna be a ho3 😩😂🙋💅," involved Chrissy dancing sensuously to Rihanna's hit song "Work" (featuring Drake). The camera slowly panned to show her wife in the background, looking unimpressed and casually scrolling her phone. The caption's emoji signal that this was a joke, with the OK symbol—having not yet been co-opted by hate groups[6]—indicating that her wife was not actually annoyed. She assumed that her viewers would identify with this common experience of unreciprocated flirting.

Chrissy asserted that emphasizing commonality was the key to attracting viewers, "If things are not relatable and you're like, very vain about what you're posting, people are not going to really care because it has nothing to do with them." Media scholar Akane Kanai (2019) defines relatability as building relationships through affect, which is "produced through labour that reflects a desirable notion of common experience to an unknown audience" (p. 4). She observes that relatability involves sharing personal experiences in ways that assume their wider generalizability. Across interviews, it became evident that this personal sharing, often as expressions of sexual identity and related relationships, communicated intimacy while the commonality established with LGBTQ viewers generated affect to spark a relationship between an individual and their audience. As Chrissy notes, others can see themselves in her skits and jokes.

In Tobias Raun's (2018) pivotal work on transgender vloggers, he identifies that the affective labor of microcelebrity relies on intimacy "as genre and as capital" (p. 100). As genre, intimacy carries a specific aesthetic derived from cultural norms, technological affordances, and platform regulation. Chrissy's joke video built on cultural norms relating to relationships, within Vine's affordances that enable the delivery of affective intensity through 6.5-second videos and the platform's tolerance of sensual dancing in its governance policies. Intimacy as genre translates into capital when it garners attention as a brand and when individuals align themselves with the sale of (often branded) commodities (Raun,

2018). As Chrissy's video received engagement in the form of views, likes, and re-Vines (shares), it appeared alongside her other Vines showcasing her wares for sale.

Another way sexual identity featured in intimate affective labor was through flirting and sexual poses as displays of queer, female desire. "Goodnight Instagram," Kelzz captioned a flirty selfie one evening. Also in her midtwenties and African American, she was working in a warehouse and hoped that her Instagram following could help her to quit in pursuit of a career as a professional dancer. Her flirting complemented the suave dance moves in her other videos, cultivating a growing fandom demonstrated by her followers' overwhelming response to a meme she posted that read, "Double-tap if you'd date me" (double-tapping is a gesture that adds a "like" to an Instagram photo). Similarly, Alex crafted photos while imagining "the cute girl I'm talking to [over Instagram], which isn't always the same cute girl but whatever one at the time." As an early twenties, gender nonconforming individual of mixed Hawaiian, Chinese, Filipino and white background, Alex was also looking to Instagram for a career boost, working as a barista while launching a clothing line for androgynous fashion. Alex was US based but looking to reach buyers internationally. Flirting through a personal account held the possibility of attracting followers who might then click on the clothing line's linked account. The propensity for sexual displays to bring people together generates what sociologist Jason Orne (2017) calls "naked intimacy" (p. 41): interpersonal connections produced through sexual and personal exchanges that are often marginalized, punished, or rendered invisible in other contexts. Although queer women's desire is often obscured in broadcast media and other public spheres, these individuals exercised agency in representing their desires. At the same time, they mimicked the prominent influencer tactic of "sex baiting," dropping hints and infusing content with the promise of sexual subject matter as a form of clickbait, luring others to engage further with their content (Abidin & Cover, 2019).

In these instances, modulating the salience of sexual identity was key to generating intimacy, produced through the disclosure of an aspect of identity presumed to be personal. It was also central to fostering affect, as embodied and emotional responses to mutual recognition between creators and their LGBTQ audiences. Since maintaining relationships with a niche audience is focal to microcelebrity (Marwick, 2016; Senft, 2008), intimate affective labor initiates this relationship with others who identify with these posts, either as imagined recipients of desire or through common experience.

Catching the attention of a niche audience, however, relies on aesthetic displays and techniques that send and boost recognizable signals of identity, modulating salience and reach together. Hashtags comprised a useful shorthand for identifying oneself as part of Instagram and Vine's nonheterosexual demographic. Broad identity labels like #lesbian or #gay retain popularity on Instagram because they allow individuals to rapidly convey a legible sexual identity, recognizable to a networked volume of users (Herrera, 2017). For Alex, hashtagging was a no-brainer: "If I feel like I look really gay, I probably will use #gay just, again, it's a big part of my identity." Since these platforms allowed several hashtags per post, individuals often combined them to communicate subsets of identity. Mïta, a white French Canadian transwoman in her midthirties, used #translesbian alongside #lesbian with the reasoning that "#lesbian is such a big cloud . . . that's when you have to get into the multiple hashtags . . . to kind of filter people, like, to funnel people that are similar to you." While #lesbian circulated her content to a larger number of users, #translesbian allowed her to self-identify more granularly and to connect with transwomen. This reach was important to her, as a wife, parent, and mature student looking to make connections in her university program and community. She circulated posts that generated both affect and intimacy, sometimes through displays of sexual desirability but more often through endearing photos of her family. The hashtags she added supported her aim to let others know "there can be two women that can have a family." She reasserted, "There can be two women that can have kids, genetic kids, you know what I mean?" Her posts countered the paucity of representations of lesbian and trans families. Some women combined sexual identity hashtags with those relating to other facets of identity, such as Chrissy's use of Black and LGBTQ hashtags to circulate her videos to other Black, queer women. Though, likely due to the smaller number of Vine users and the relatively large volume of queer female users, there was less diversity in hashtags on this platform, with women often posting under broader LGBTQ phrases like #LGBTCrew, #RainbowGang, and #AllQueerHere.

Hashtags also helped in the promotion of one's work and career. As a tattoo artist, Emi received training from the tattoo shop manager: "She literally made us a list of, like, "These are the hashtags you should use for your tattoos here," and I literally copy and paste almost the same hashtags into every single photo that I do for tattoos and then I'll add a few." The use of Instagram for work and additional coaching from Queenie, who had "a bazillion" more followers, contributed to Emi's promotion of drag king performances, adding #dragkingsofinstagram to photos taken at shows. However, Emi still often deferred to Queenie's expertise, mumbling that understanding hashtags better was a recent development: "I was like, 'why are people putting this stupid number mark before everything?'" The effort of finding hashtags with enough uptake to make them useful, paired with their skillful deployment on relevant posts, constitutes labor contributing to effective self-branding.

While hashtags circulate posts, sexual identity is integrated into the content of photos and videos according to aesthetic practices and recognizable references to LGBTQ culture. Thea, a white Australian graduate student in her late twenties, tailored her Instagram selfies to align with what she saw others do while subtly indicating her sexual identity through fashion. Gazing at what she described as a "very staged photo" of her reading on a rainy day, she admitted to posting it because she liked how she looked in her backwards hat, which was "a lesbian thing." She explained, "I wear a lot of backwards hats to, sort of, make a statement to people who—because I don't—because I think I look straight, so it sort of lets people know . . . other lesbians are going to know, generally." Popularized by queer female celebrities and influencers, such as Thea's favorite influencer Hannah Hart, the backwards hat has become well established among lesbian fashion tropes. Thea couched this display of lesbian fashion within common elements of Instagram style, including soft lighting, views of home decor, and documenting one's self-improvement, such as by reading lauded novels.

Similar to how queer women in chapter 2 signaled their sexual identity on Tinder, interview participants across Instagram and Vine sampled from a recognizable menu of stereotypes and tropes, combined with their individual flare, to communicate queer aesthetic as part of a personal brand. When discussing style choices, Alex declared, "The more I look like Justin Bieber in the pictures, the better," signaling a gay identity through a short, Bieber-style haircut, which was popular among queer women in the mid-2010s (evidenced by Tumblr blogs with titles like "Lesbians who look like Justin Bieber"). Backwards hats and Bieber haircuts play with gender expression and displays of feminine masculinity in ways that have long signaled nonheterosexuality (Brickman, 2016).

These aesthetic displays, and the ability to circulate them to wider audiences, rely on the development of skills and techniques. Kamala, a Thai lesbian in her early forties, posted beautiful landscapes to inspire her followers. Earlier in life, she was diagnosed with lupus and became very ill, but upon her recovery she wanted to share her insights by becoming a motivational speaker. She aimed to foster audiences for her speaking events through Instagram. Her photos showcased many perspectives on one location to captivate followers visually, enhancing visibility through hashtags relevant to lupus survivors and lesbians as combined facets of her identity. Julie, a white Canadian children's program facilitator in her late forties, also sought to create captivating images and flaunted her photo-editing skills: "I can make any photo Instagram-worthy. . . . If it's a flattering picture, I'm like, 'Oh, I look good in this picture, let's bring it—I can tweak this picture.'" She rose to Instagram's invocation to turn images into art by using filters and manual editing features. With Vine's dearth of editing tools, Chrissy banded with fellow Viners to find a third-party app for adding music to videos. By the time Vine rolled out an update with a similar feature, she felt it was redundant: "[Vine] took forever to get on our level when we've been doing it, so it doesn't even matter." Such behind-the-scenes strategies and modifications enhanced these women's display of their intimate affective content.

However, these approaches take time to learn and effort to develop. Several women admitted they did not fully understand certain app features. Julie revealed the trial-and-error process of selecting hashtags for her business, having tried many variations of hashtags to promote her latest children's yoga program. She sighed, "Nobody has said to me, 'Hey, I was searching for kids' programs and I came across you.'" Similarly, Kelzz noted troubles with Instagram's automatic photo sizing, "I still get cut off sometimes with some of my pictures." In her study of established Singaporean influencers, Crystal Abidin (2016) identifies that their bodily comportment, makeup, and fashion, as well as technology and editing skills, constitute tacit labor as "a collective practice of work that is understated and under-visibilized from being so thoroughly rehearsed that it appears effortless and subconscious" (p. 10). While some women I spoke with applied techniques that appeared effortless, much of their developmental aesthetic labor was evident, and not tacit, in the training that participants underwent, advice they sought from others, and the occasional cut-off photo or poorly timed song.

Training and experience were fundamental for transforming developmental into tacit labor. Jaxx, an American Viner in her early twenties who had the largest following of anyone I spoke with, accrued more than twenty thousand followers through her comedic skits about being Latina, bisexual, and neurodivergent.[7] She spoke casually about the aesthetics of her videos: "I look back [and] I'm like, 'Damn, I probably should have fixed my eyeliner. I probably should have worn a t-shirt.'" Jaxx tended to wake up in the middle of the night, inspired by an idea, and commence filming without putting on a shirt or doing her makeup. For this reason, several of her videos depict her as a talking head with bare shoulders, bringing a literal sense to Orne's (2017) concept of "naked intimacy" mentioned earlier. She continued: "I've had people tell me like, 'Yo, your confidence and the fact that you really don't care has helped me to do that.' So, should I think about how I set up my Vines? Probably. Do I? No. I mean, sometimes it's because, again, a lot of my inspiration is improv because that's what I was taught back at theater school. . . . It's off the top of your head." While her approach reflected Vine's affordances for sharing spontaneous, unedited footage, she also described a refined and increasingly common aesthetic: the art of not caring. As the influencer industry has grown, Abidin (2018) observes that "calibrated amateurism" has become a common form of labor "crafting contrived authenticity that portrays the raw aesthetic of an amateur" (p. 91) regardless of whether one really is an amateur. This labor, which requires honing one's self-representational skills, gives followers the sense that they are accessing real and authentic glimpses of a person's life. Jaxx's mention of previous training in improvisation and theater, potentially enhanced by her day job in marketing, underscores the developmental work that occurred prior to her Vine debut. This enabled her to move from developmental aesthetic labor to the seamless application of more tacit forms of labor, including calibrated amateurism.

Aspiring Relational Labor

Several women I spoke with endeavored to forge ongoing and potentially lucrative relationships with figures who resonated with their followers. They often tried to grab the attention of popular users with large follower counts by "shouting out" to them: tagging them in a photo or caption. This was done in hopes the individual would *shout* back at them, directing followers' attention to their account. Alex experienced this reciprocity when connecting with a transgender Instagrammer who had thousands of followers and his own clothing line for nonbinary, transgender, and gender-nonconforming people: "[He] shouted out my account on his personal page and it just blew up, so I ended up asking him to come in as the co-owner and he really made things take off. Within a month, I had reached my goal of one thousand followers." Alex asked the Instagrammer to help manage the androgynous clothing line's account. Such follower sharing and mentorship is common among influencers, such as when YouTubers make guest appearances on others' channels or Instagrammers forge "pods" based on collective agreements to boost each other's engagement (Abidin, 2018; Morris & Anderson, 2015).

Some women I interviewed also understood these platforms as making it possible to connect with celebrities through avenues that did not exist previously. In vetting her Vine content, Jaxx considered how it might be viewed through celebrity eyes: "Look, if Ellen DeGeneres finds my Vine and I happened to use the wrong word when I was ignorant and stupid— I'm very conscious about how people are going to read it." As one of the few celebrities on Vine, DeGeneres had the capacity to endow Viners with fame as she regularly spotlighted them on her daytime talk show.[8] Making this scenario of overnight discovery a reality, Kelzz was pleased to win a celebrity's dance contest and have one of her videos appear on their Instagram page. With the celebrity's large fan base, she observed that her video would "reach somebody who has zero followers to somebody who has fifteen thousand followers," circulating well beyond her immediate audience. Similarly, Alex's sales surged when the clothing account was tagged in a notable photo: "There was a picture of Ruby Rose holding a pair of my boxers that came out, and I sold a few hundred pairs that week." Thanks to Rose's status as an icon of androgynous fashion, the image of her holding a pair of Alex's branded underwear sparked fans' interest and investment.

These efforts reinforce Duffy's (2016) observation that forming instrumental relationships is a key component of aspirational labor. She identifies how aspirational beauty and fashion bloggers pour affective labor into maintaining relationships with peers and audiences on platforms while also establishing relationships in person, such as at networking events. The women I spoke with also conducted this affective labor, responding to follower comments and liking others' posts. Queenie recalled one of several instances when this relationship maintenance carried over in person: "We went to a roller derby event Saturday night and one of the roller girls came up to me and said, 'Oh my God, [Queenie], I stalk you on Instagram.'" She marveled at her account's reach: "I feel like, especially locally, I have a really great exposure to people through Instagram." But beyond the general maintenance of follower relationships, participants strived to form relationships with popular users from a preexisting state of uneven status. Sociologist Forrest Stuart (2020) reveals that Black youth music creators who achieve social media fame often deal with the problem of fans latching on to them for the purpose of "clouting up" (p. 107). Those with an established following accumulated "clout"—a reputation of notoriety and a following—and those clouting up aimed to feature in their videos or find other ways to share in these young people's microcelebrity. I view these efforts, whether shouting out, looking to be featured, or tailoring content to attract popular users' attention, as a subset of aspirational labor that aims toward the relational—hence the phrase "aspiring relational labor"— in recognition that "relational labor has the potential to bring both revenue and meaningful connection" (Baym, 2018, p. 28). Taking the leap to reach out to someone with much clout who does not know you exist can have great returns, but that individual needs a reason to take notice.

Participants understood meaningful connection as being possible not only through platform features that increased their reach but specifically through the display of sexual identity as a common ground on which to form relationships. Jaxx imagined that her witty bisexual jokes would make Ellen DeGeneres laugh, while Alex's clothing brand resonated with the popular Instagrammer's gender-related activism. Influencers often perform unpaid product promotion—raving about a brand they absolutely *love*—and tailor their content to align with brand campaigns in hopes of gaining sponsorships (Carter, 2016; Duffy, 2016). Aspiring relational labor, comprised of such efforts to attract the attention of popular users and retain it through shared nonheterosexual identity, resembles this sort of "hustling" (Carter, 2016), where the brand being touted is sexual identity. However, these individuals strived to connect with people, whereas commercial brands and products were tangential or subsequent to their interpersonal relationship building. Further, they perceived their focus on shared identity would be well-received, poten- tially creating a lasting and genuine bond and contrasting starkly with the shallow connotations attached to doing something for the hustle or using someone for their clout.

The three forms of labor I have described are overlapping and mutually reinforcing. For example, aesthetic displays can channel intimacy, affect, and a sense of shared likeness if executed effectively. Overall, they resemble common microcelebrity practices: carrying out affective labor to connect with a niche audience, implementing skills to produce content according to platform and audience norms, and maintaining relationships with others who could instrumentally contribute to one's success. However, the reconceptualization of these practices into labor involving identity modu- lation captures the effort that these queer women made to integrate sexual identity into their self-branding, especially in early stages of building status on these platforms. Through their interaction with platform affordances for extending reach, these women tailored the salience of sexual identity in their self-representations to garner greater attention through efforts toward circulating affectively intimate content, formulating aesthetically resonant displays, and establishing powerful relationships with popular individuals.

Although the women I interviewed often engaged in these modes of labor with the intention of expanding their reach, they exercised volume control, grappling with modulating reach according to specific audiences and in tandem with their personal identifiability. Choosing to have a public, rather than private, account on Instagram depended on some women's comfort with extending their reach to unknown audiences. Emi created an Instagram account based on the suspicion that Facebook rarely surfaced unpaid posts showcasing tattoo work in people's News Feeds. Emi scoffed at the idea of having a private account, "Well, what's the point of doing it if—how do you get all this attention for things if only the people I select see it? Kind of defeats the purpose." While being public allowed Emi to reach potential, previously unknown clients, the combination of tattoos, couple selfies, and posts reflecting sexual identity had an unexpected outcome: it piqued the interest of queer people who preferred a queer tattoo artist and weeded out homophobic potential clients.

In contrast, Julie struggled constantly with how to modulate her account's reach in relation to the salience of her sexual identity due to the nature of her work. Specializing in children's programming, she felt a duty to protect the youth she worked with from "creepy people" and opted to post photos of herself, rather than the children in her recreational programs, showcasing daily routines of planning and setting up for work but also including snapshots from her personal life. Although Julie was not secretive about being married to her wife, she found it important to be subtle about their relationship in photos because her programs were often associated with a Christian church. As she scrolled through her account, she pointed out a photo collage with a small image of her and her partner kissing and laughingly described it as "the most outrageous thing I've done on social media!" But she became somber as she explained that making her sexual identity more visible "could pose a threat potentially, especially with children. People might say things like, 'I don't want you to turn my kids gay.'" She chose to extend the reach of her account and, in turn, people's knowledge of her children's programs while downplaying the salience of her sexual identity.

These contrasting examples illustrate enduring perceptions and biases related to identity and labor. Namely, they reflect ideas about who is fit to do a certain kind of job. In some instances, nonheterosexual identity may be congruent with an occupational persona, especially in occupations that are often linked to subcultures or countercultures, such as tattooing or burlesque. However, Julie's experience attests to certain occupations remaining firmly tied to unsubstantiated traditional or religious notions, such as the idea that people can *turn* children gay as though sexuality were contagious. As feminist scholar Sara Ahmed (2006) writes with regard to enduring lines of inheritance, children are often raised with the assumption that they will grow up to extend the family line through a heteronormative family formation. Ahmed plays with the notion of lines to illustrate how entrenched these perceptions remain, identifying how an assumed line of inheritance is like a well-trodden path formed through repetition, which endures as it has become the easiest way to travel through life. Deviating from that path takes considerable effort and is highly noticeable. Careers or occupations can be inherited in that they traverse generations that imbue them with expectations about how duties should be fulfilled and by whom. Teaching and child care—elements of Julie's job—in particular have been associated with (often unpaid) women's labor and serve to support entrenched social and economic structures, including the heteronormative nuclear family. Thus, it makes sense that Julie views the occasional photo displaying affection toward her wife as radical in her line of work.

Potential clients and homophobic strangers were not the only audiences who concerned the women I interviewed. For several, building a self-brand that included displays of sexual identity on these specific platforms helped to manage whether and how this content appeared to family, friends, and acquaintances. Jaxx and Chrissy drew on Vine's affordances to channel broad audiences that excluded offline acquaintances through the use of pseudonyms and thanks to Vine's relatively smaller uptake in contrast to other platforms. Interviewees using Instagram similarly relied on its separation from Facebook, a platform where many maintained different audiences. Alex posted sexually themed content to Instagram with the rationale, "My grandma is on Facebook but she's not on Instagram, so I'm OK with posting it on Instagram because no one I'm related to is going to see it. . . . Facebook is more family oriented." Although user demographics are not static, Instagram has been known to attract a younger user population, with 67 percent of Americans ages eighteen to twenty-nine on the platform in 2019, compared to only 23 percent of those ages fifty to sixty-four (Perrin & Monica, 2019). This age separation was pronounced for Kamala, who was in her forties and reflected on being an outlier, "My Facebook friends and Facebook followers don't like to use Instagram."

Unlike on Vine, many of the women on Instagram posted content rendering them easily recognizable to offline acquaintances, sometimes even adopting usernames representative of their legal names. This higher level of identifiability follows platform norms that have evolved over time with Instagram's increasing use for self-promotion and the transfer of expectations from Facebook to Instagram (Leaver, 2015). Individuals often clearly displayed their faces and other identifiers, such as their homes, with the awareness that posts could be found by others with whom they would not normally share these self-representations. Mïta acknowledged, "There are pictures on Instagram that are a little more risqué." She scrolled through images that included a selfie in which she was posing in a swimsuit, "Like, there's more boob-age or whatever, and having my grandparents or uncles and aunts on [Facebook]—it's like, if they want to see it, they can go on my Instagram, you know what I mean?" She stressed that she was not trying to hide these images or keep them private, as they were a source of pride, reflecting her satisfaction with her body after transitioning, and her followers found them inspirational. However, she did not want to push them into her family's view, as Facebook's News Feed algorithm was known to do indiscriminately. For Mïta and several participants, Instagram served as a *pull* platform, which could garner the attention of widespread audiences while requiring those who wished to regularly view content to take the necessary steps to access Instagram, find their account, and follow it. This differed from Facebook, where participation was often felt as requisite due to its popularity and friend requests were normatively accepted, resulting in images being *pushed* by the platform to accumulated audiences of family and friends who might bristle at sexual or identity-related content not intended for them.

Despite these women's intentional separation of Instagram and Vine from other social media, the platforms included design features to bridge these gaps. Vine urged users to connect their Twitter accounts and import followers. Instagram went one step further to make accumulating the same contacts across platforms seamless by notifying users when their Facebook friends also joined Instagram. Thea, who was not out to all her friends and family, experienced face-palm moments revealing the futility of her painstaking steps to maintain her Instagram content separate from Facebook, disabling cross-platform posting and self-censoring Facebook posts by removing lesbian content. People commonly told her, "I found you on Instagram because I had you on Facebook." This platform-initiated context collapse made her wary of posting about sexual identity at all.

CONCLUSION: WHO PROFITS FROM THE PERSONAL?

This chapter has explored what identity modulation looks like when channeled into platformed practices of self-branding. Identity modulation featured in multiple modes of labor through which queer women harnessed Instagram's aesthetically pleasing filters, Vine's looping videos, and other platform features to circulate content displaying sexual identity as part of a personal brand. In amplifying sexual identity, these women aimed to generate intimacy and affect among followers, target LGBTQ market niches through resonant signals and aesthetics, and communicate a common ground for connecting with well-established users and celebrities. This labor of putting themselves *out there* was paired with modulating personal identifiability and the salience of sexual identity to build a self-brand among intended, potentially lucrative audiences. Their identity modulation also included efforts to maintain other audiences as separate, particularly those with whom this branded persona did not accord or was unnecessary, such as family members who were unlikely clients or fans.

On Instagram and Vine, queer women understood platform metrics (e.g., likes, shares, followers) as indicators of whether their labor was successful. Kelzz described this evidence of engagement as "my pusher—it tells me to keep going." Interviewees reflexively responded to metrics, adjusting their self-representations according to follower responses. However, Queenie expressed frustration with this feedback loop: "Anything that's slightly sexual or nudity-wise is the stuff that blows up. And because of that, I absolutely do it and use it to my benefit but," she sighed, "I just think it's super tragic that those are the ones that get promoted all over the place when I feel like I have stuff that means a lot more that doesn't go that far." While her burlesque dancing and associated brand incorporated sexual and semi-nude displays, she also wished her political and activist content would gain comparable attention. Although the axiom of "sex sells" may lead us to conclude that sexual images will always attract the greatest engagement, attempts to boost metrics also involve negotiating platform algorithms that determine which content is widely circulated and how it ranks in others' feeds (Bucher, 2012; Gillespie, 2012). Investigators allege that Instagram's algorithm prioritizes photos of women in swimwear or underwear in users' feeds over other kinds of content, concluding that the algorithm skews toward displaying and circulating (semi-)nudity (Duportail et al., 2020). A lack of transparency about how the algorithm functions makes it impossible to know whether this skew is intentional, an outcome of user practices, or merely a byproduct of machine-learning techniques Instagram may be using. Regardless, individuals learn to tailor their content to appease not only followers but also platform requirements for visibility (Bishop, 2018).

Vying for engagement among selective algorithms and followers' limited attentional capacity demands that individuals remain fresh and competitive. By the time I interviewed Chrissy in 2016, users had begun leaving Vine in droves, and she told me, "Vine is completely broken." She explained that the platform showcased a small concentration of users while others found it difficult to gain any attention for their videos. She evaluated the situation: "Either you're Vine famous or you're not and that's just it." Features that elevated select users and rampant competition to become "Vine famous" generated animosity while contributing to a homogeneity of content. With few creators gaining brand sponsorships from their Vine notoriety and no clear path for monetizing content, many up-and-coming users quit shortly before Vine was decommissioned in early 2017 (Lorenz, 2016). Chrissy, who found the competition exhausting and petty, was already disengaging from the platform when we spoke. For a while, Vine's competitiveness had spurred users to generate volumes of content, supporting Terranova's (2000) observation that users sustain the value of digital properties. However, this competitive atmosphere eventually backfired for Vine when it led to creators' departure.

Pressure on individual creators to make a name for themselves and to produce content with impressive metrics can also lead to a sense of exploitation and estrangement from one's personal sharing. After Jaxx's Vines were featured in the app's comedy section, a representative from Twitter (Vine's parent company) reached out to say, "The company's aware of who you are." The representative provided tips for gaining followers and encouraged Jaxx to make more videos, especially since she intervened in the white, male-dominated scene of top Viners. Although this interaction did not come with the promise of tangible reward, Jaxx felt that it added pressure to her creative process: "I just feel like, especially talking to this lady, it's gotten me very overly aware of my Vines. And now when I try to do Vines, my improv isn't coming as fluidly because I'm starting to care and I'm starting to think, 'Shit, is it funny?' and 'Shit, is this going to get the loop count?'" That Jaxx ticked the *diversity* box for Vine laid bare how her production was about boosting engagement for the platform with relatively little payoff for her, which led to feelings of insecurity and exploitation.

Further, Jaxx started to feel estranged from her content: "The moment it starts feeling like a job—like a chore—it's not fun anymore, and it's no longer authentically myself." Since her Vines shared personal and, in turn, intimate aspects of her identity, deploying these as labor within the context of (potential) economic exchange made their content feel contrived. Sociologist Christian Fuchs and media scholar Nick Dyer-Witheford (2013) remind us that long-standing Marxist principles still apply to digital economies. They identify that internet studies often uncover worker alienation, as users' labor power is appropriated for platforms' capitalist means, eventuating in users having little control or ownership over what they produce. Vine benefited from Jaxx's labor as she produced fresh content that broke up the platform's homogeneity while she began to feel distanced from her personal, creative outputs.

Labor arrangements within the digital economy also pose the risk of individuals being seen as selling out, projecting an identity for the sole purpose of profit. The commercialization of LGBTQ identities is often at odds with their political efficacy. Queer social media influencers face this tension as they attempt to monetize a following gained through their representation of LGBTQ lives, politics, and activism (Raun, 2018). Indeed, the women I interviewed often incorporated generic LGBTQ indicators of identity in ways that seem to support Michael Lovelock's (2017) concern that social media celebrities' "practices of authenticity, self-branding and self-revelation" (p. 93) reinforce the representation of homonormative identities. But their self-brands also garnered followings of people who felt they were relatable, helped to weed out homophobic clients, and—as we will see in chapter 4—attracted both platform censorship and heterosexist, misogynist harassment. If these women's personal displays constituted mere homonormative representations, devoid of impact due to mainstream reproduction and commercialization, they would be unlikely to invoke such responses.

A growing subset of microcelebrity literature identifies how LGBTQ influencers are attempting to balance the communities they convene through genuine personal sharing with the need to make a living from their labor (Abidin & Cover, 2019; Cunningham & Craig, 2017; Raun, 2018). Raun (2018) observes that the intimate disclosures of Julie Van Vu, a transgender vlogger, are the glue that retains her loyal fans even as she increasingly features advertorials on her YouTube channel. Similarly, Abidin and Cover (2019) identify that queer influencers encounter opportunities for activism alongside branded sponsorships. This balance is comparable for some of the queer women I interviewed, whom I have seen move into more public roles as queer performers, entertainers, and creators as they continue to showcase their personal lives and increase their potentially monetizable followings.

Overall, the experiences recounted in this chapter show that the labor of identity modulation is not *only* exploited by platforms as part of their user-reliant profit models, nor is it exploitation free. A million-dollar smile is at the mercy of platform algorithms and metrics as well as features that complicate volume control, all while platforms stand to profit from content generated through identity modulation. At the same time, platform affordances for amplifying reach hold promise for increasing ordinary people's social and economic participation, especially in individualized fields of work where affective intimacy, resonant aesthetics, and powerful relationships are integral to success. A cute photo hashtagged #lesbehonest may simultaneously inspire followers while running the risk of being cliché, but at the end of the day, it fulfills social media's increasing demand for identity-based self-branding.

CHAPTER 4

Beyond the Gated Community

Salience in Publics and Counterpublics

I n the 1990s, sociologist Nina Wakeford (1996) brought us into the world of a listserv named "Sappho." Listservs are electronic mailing lists, which often allow for threaded conversation among subscribers. Since Sappho was a subscriber-only list for lesbian- and bisexual-identified women, one could only be added by sending the "list mistress" a message specifying one's gender as female. Once added, participants were further vetted by others, who inferred details of a woman's gender expression and sexual preferences through her writing style and topics of choice. "Sapphites," as Wakeford called them, brought further information about their personal qualities into dialogue through signature blocks with links to homepages or lyrics by queer female artists, such as k. d. lang, and text pertaining to the Muff Diva Index (MDI). The MDI was a coded set of labels enabling individuals to indicate their place on a number of scales relating to femme-butch gender expression, hair length, heels versus sneakers, and other dimensions of desirability and personality common to—or stereotypical of—lesbian and bisexual women's self-expression. Such identity codes were prone to change over time, but Wakeford underscores that they were refashioned communally. This personal sharing and collective identity construction facilitated intimate conversations among women on the listserv, sharing views that "might not necessarily be spoken elsewhere" and thus giving rise to the "feeling of being 'home'" and among family (p. 101).

Reflecting on the Sappho listserv allows for comparison across identity signaling practices, their outcomes, and the affordances of different digital

Personal but Not Private. Stefanie Duguay, Oxford University Press. © Oxford University Press 2022.
DOI: 10.1093/oso/9780190076184.003.0004

contexts. Collective identity signaling was observed on early websites and forums, such as in gay men's gatherings on Usenet (O'Riordan, 2005) and in the Lesbian Cafe, a bulletin board service that Shelley Correll (1995) studied. Mary L. Gray's (2009) groundbreaking work on LGBTQ rural youth identified their collective labor of crafting and articulating queer identity across websites and Facebook as well as in their small towns. These young people determined what *queer* looked like apart from the dominant expressions cultivated in, and exported from, progressive metropolises. With such collective identity work, not everyone claims the same identity or expresses a common identity in similar ways—not all women on Sappho identified as femme, for example—but there is a collective understanding and recognition of potential connection stemming from a shared identity and its relation to the rest of society. For self-identified LGBTQ people, we must make sense of what this identity means for us as well as how its social, cultural, and historical definition may shape our (and others') interpretations of this identity. Therefore, people find connection in how they define themselves and through common experiences of how others treat them as a result of this identity.

Social media platforms shift the context for this collective identity work. Chat rooms and listservs that vet their members through identity displays can be understood as gated communities of sorts, with informal and sometimes formal mechanisms of keeping out those who do not identify in similar ways. Popular platforms instead see uptake from a range of users, resulting in heterogeneity that presents the potential for a wider diversity of people to convene in dialogue. However, this heterogeneity also complicates how individuals with similar identifications find each other and stake out space for bonding, establishing representation, and making identity-based statements.

In response, individuals can remediate offline cultural practices, imbuing them with digital elements that enhance their recognizability within a platform context. Critical race scholars André Brock (2012, 2020) and Sarah Florini (2014) observe this process in their work on Black Twitter. Florini describes the Black cultural practice of "signifyin'" as a "linguistic performance that allows for the communication of multiple levels of meaning simultaneously, most frequently involving wordplay and misdirection" (p. 224). Signifyin' melds with Twitter's hashtags, tweet character limit, and conventions of public display to give rise to a new technocultural practice—one that is a hybrid of cultural expression and digital affordances. In relation to this practice, which would not exist without the platform, Brock (2012) asserts that "Black hashtag signifying revealed alternate Twitter discourses to the mainstream and encourages a formulation of Black

Twitter as a 'social public'; a community constructed through their use of social media by outsiders and insiders alike" (p. 530). A sense of community can be generated through such technocultural practices, which tend to include signals of shared identifications. This community sense resembles the family-like feeling on Sappho, except social publics on platforms are generally accessible to onlookers, who may or may not understand, condone, or support the group identity being expressed.

In this chapter, I return to the everyday collective identity signals of queer women on Instagram and Vine, which indicate the formation of social publics among them. This analysis allows for an understanding of how such publics are constructed, the functions they serve, and what they may or may not accomplish within platform constraints. Since danah boyd's (2014) conceptualization of networked publics as publics "restructured by networked technologies" (p. 8), several scholars have identified different kinds of networked publics arising from specific arrangements of what boyd describes as the "intersection of people, technology, and practice" (p. 8). To understand these elaborations, it is helpful to revisit certain cornerstone theorizations of the public sphere. Boyd (2011) highlights feminist theorist Nancy Fraser's critique of philosopher Jürgen Habermas's vision of a unitary public sphere, which assumes that differences can be bracketed, or put aside, to deliberate issues as equals. By bracketing differences, Habermas envisions these discussions taking place among men with a similar status to himself, thus excluding women and other individuals whose participation in society is already limited by inequality or discrimination. These individuals, who are marked by their differences and therefore cannot bracket them, are omitted from this vision of the public sphere on account of their personal matters being deemed private issues to be dealt with away from public view. However, Fraser (1990) argues that personal matters must feature in publics to invoke social change. She points out that, rather than one public sphere, multiple overlapping publics exist, including "subaltern counterpublics" that develop and circulate counterdiscourses. Subaltern counterpublics function "as spaces of withdrawal and regroupment" as well as "bases and training grounds for agitational activities directed toward wider publics" (p. 68). Put another way, subaltern counterpublics provide solidarity from which to challenge the status quo.

Literary scholars Michael Warner and Lauren Berlant highlight the relevance of texts—forms of discourse ranging from speech to books, film, and other media—in shaping publics. Warner (2002) defines publics as organized around discourse and, dropping "subaltern," identifies that counterpublics often produce their own texts, as they function in a state of tension with larger publics. In their analysis of American "women's culture," Berlant (2008) identifies an intimate public formed through women's construction in, and response to, texts identifying them as consumers with shared interests and desires. Placing these concepts within digital contexts, social media posts often serve as texts with the potential to gather publics. Networked intimate publics (Olszanowski, 2014) reflect connections that can form in relation to intimate content circulating through hashtags while networked counterpublics (Renninger, 2015) gravitate to counterdiscourses shared through community-building platform features. This chapter takes a close look at the interplay between personal—but shared—identity practices and platform affordances to identify queer women's emergent publics.

The salience of sexual identity in queer women's collective identity work gives rise to these platform-specific publics. Identity modulation, on the part of the user and the platform, leads to variable degrees of salience that shape a public's intensity and reception among other users. Platforms play a key role in shaping shared engagement with focal texts—generally, user posts—and the interactions this engagement may spark with others. With Tinder serving up profiles for users to vet individually and facilitating only one-on-one matching and chatting, users do not congregate around profiles or any other content on this platform in a way that could concretely be thought of as a public.[1] Consequently, queer women on Tinder are stuck with the lesbian digital imaginary, discussed in chapter 2, that allows them to conceive of a broader community of nonheterosexual women on the app but does not give rise to collective exchanges. Digital imaginaries are not anchored through social interactions in the same way as publics. As such, Tinder did not emerge as a locus for queer women's publics and counterpublics in my research.

Instead, this chapter focuses on platforms conducive to broader dialogue and content circulation. On Instagram, practices of polished and commercial self-branding enable the formation of an intimate public that is fairly benign in its politics but gives the impression that the "good life" (Berlant, 2008) of neoliberal citizenship is available to young queer women. Instagram's commercially oriented, heavily homonormative collective identity signaling contrasts with the intimate and often sexual posts queer women circulated on Vine, which facilitated close-knit communities and the formation of a counterpublic perpetuated through videos challenging heterosexism alongside racism, ableism, and other oppressive biases. However, the collective salience of their sexual identity makes queer women on social media a target for those who aim to censor, harass, and discriminate. The experiences women shared with me underscore that it is perilous to leave gated communities. Not only do platforms' governance policies, and their associated design features, fail to protect marginalized identity groups, they also enable targeting and harassment that constrain vulnerable users' social media participation and can lead them to drop out of publics altogether.

INSTAGRAM'S FANTASY PUBLIC

As I scrolled through hundreds of Instagram photos posted to queer women's hashtags in 2015, I spotted a repeating figure. She was tall, slim, and generally light-skinned, though she sometimes appeared on the beach with a tan. She often eschewed heavy makeup for minimal eyeliner, and her hair was usually long and straight, draping across her shoulders under a backwards hat or toque. This woman donned mostly feminine clothing with a masculine accessory or twist to queer her look: a sports jacket, a plaid button-up, a skateboard or sneakers. She traipsed across beautiful landscapes and urban scenes in photos with filters applied to make the light fuzzy, fragmented, and almost mystical. Her images appeared with the most popular queer women's hashtags like #lesbiansofinstagram and #girlswholikegirls, often depicting her embracing or kissing another woman who possessed similar features, as though she were making out with herself.

Of course, I am not merely describing one woman. This fantastical trope was prominent across queer women's hashtags and, while the individual women in these images were distinguishable upon closer inspection, I was struck by their overall similarity. These women tended to resemble mainstream representations of queer women in film and television, who are still generally played by young, thin, white, and feminine actors more than anyone else (Smith & Tyler, 2017).

Instead of being traceable to a particular user, these images were often shared by aggregator accounts, those created with the purpose of reposting others' content and aggregating it around a certain theme or hashtag. Accounts were often run by self-proclaimed teenagers, with multiple "owners" listed in their biographies. The affinity of presumably young, queer women for these idealized photos resonates with a practice that feminist scholar Amy Dobson (2015) identified among heterosexual teenage girls. She noticed that their Myspace profiles, and later their Facebook walls, were sprinkled with seductive and sexualized images of women, which she termed "digital dreamgirls." Dobson conceptualizes "heterosexy" aesthetics as those in alignment with normative standards of femininity and heteronormativity, and digital dreamgirls represent the pinnacle of heterosexiness. Commonly, digital dreamgirls included women affiliated with brands or media franchises (e.g., Paris Hilton), as commoditized media transformations and replications of the *ideal* desirable woman.

Although the digital dreamgirls that queer women shared on Instagram were not heterosexual, as proclaimed through masculine fashion items, queer hashtags, and depictions of same-sex couples, they exuded heterosexiness through their adherence to heteronormative beauty standards. They also embodied success defined in neoliberal terms through displays of affluence and homonormativity (Warner, 1999), underscored by the absence of deviations from the hegemonic idealization of white supremacy, ability, and the retention of femininity. This lesbian digital dreamgirl—and I say "lesbian" because the images lacked antinormative politics often associated with the term queer—frequently featured in picturesque wedding scenes or at honeymoon destinations, continuing the heteronormative romantic storyline of marriage leading to the formation of a nuclear family. Notably these storylines abound even on contemporary television shows featuring queer women. For example, *The L Word: Generation Q* (2019–)—a purportedly more progressive reboot of the 2000s original series about a friend group of (mostly) lesbian women (Keating, 2019)—ran multiple plotlines about marriage and childrearing in its first season. These themes are also pervasive among queer female YouTubers, with Hannah Hart featuring her engagement and subsequent search for a wedding dress while the popular couple Sam and Alyssa share their parenting experiences with subscribers. As likely audiences for this content, young queer women on Instagram appeared to be circulating and reinforcing similar themes with their likes, comments, and further sharing.

This figure of the lesbian digital dreamgirl indicated the presence of a networked intimate public of queer women on Instagram, as its manifestations constituted a prominent shared text that convened this public. Berlant (2008) underscores that publics become intimate when there is an expectation of commonality imposed upon and taken up by the public's constituents, stemming from a "broadly common historical experience" (p. viii). Popular queer women's hashtags provide one example of how individuals on Instagram claim common identities based on an assumed shared experience of being female and LGBTQ (Herrera, 2017). Intimate publics circulate texts that are intentionally fantastical and filled with hyperbole as roadmaps to "enduring, resisting, overcoming, and enjoying being an *x*" (Berlant, 2008, p. viii), where an *x* is a member of a nondominant population. The lesbian digital dreamgirl, shared through these hashtags, represented this roadmap as she displayed the "good life" (p. 9), a phrase Berlant uses to point to fantasies of neoliberal thriving. The lesbian digital dreamgirl depicted a desirable and successful female homosexual lifestyle within society's structures. This contrasts with the rejection, discrimination, and blocked access to civil rights that were often the dominant reality for gays and lesbians in the recent history of many countries and that still haunt LGBTQ youth as they share these posts imagining futures of desirability and flourishing.

Berlant (2008) defines an intimate public as foregrounded in "affective and emotional attachments located in fantasies of the common, the everyday, and a sense of ordinariness" (p. 10). While images of lesbian digital dreamgirls captured common fantasy scenes, their poses, fashion, and filtered aesthetics were recreated in queer women's everyday selfies, which dominated these hashtags. As described in the previous chapter, a great deal of developmental aesthetic labor goes into obtaining an Instagram-worthy look, which accords with Instafamous practices emulating celebrity styles (Marwick, 2015). Beyond interview participants' self-branding, I observed these broader themes across self-representational photos, which tended to showcase similar elements of the good life: happy relationships, envy-inspiring travel, stylish fashion, and commodity accessories. These images contributed to a queer women's intimate public organized around "commodity culture" (Berlant, 2008, p. 8), which responded to and perpetuated visions of LGBTQ consumer life that are widely targeted by marketers and that enable claiming identity through consumption within capitalism. The consumer aspect of this intimate public is exactly what opened up the potential for economic success through self-branding highlighted in chapter 3.

Vague Connections

Within this intimate public on Instagram, the women I interviewed both benefited from and contributed to the collective work of building and reinforcing a shared sense of queer women's identity and experience. Kelzz reflected on how her sense of self shifted after she made her account public: "It kind of broke the shell I was hiding in—in a way, and it opened me up to be even more okay about who I am." As she shared her dance videos with queer hashtags, she felt connected to a broad community whom she viewed as her motivation for creating more content. For Mïta, others' engagement with her photos helped her to feel positive about herself post-transition: "You have all this reinforcement from people who are in a similar situation commenting and liking your pictures, you know, so it's a bit of a boost there."

With these affirmations of their sense of identity, several of the women I spoke with felt motivated to give back by making their sexual identity a salient part of their self-representations and connecting with other queer women. Kamala included #lesbian on her everyday photos because people "never show about 'I am lesbian' and [what it is] to live the lesbian way in Thailand." She aimed to contribute to what she called an "LGBT world" on Instagram so that queer Thai women could see they were not alone. Mita received daily emails requesting advice about transitioning and living as a transgender lesbian. She responded to each message with the reasoning, "I was once one of those people that was struggling with how to do this, you know, so I get back to everybody that is looking for help." Through photos, hashtags, and responses to other Instagrammers, these women contributed to publics organized by particular facets of identity (e.g., lesbian, transgender) and situated within broader publics (e.g., LGBTQ users, Thai users).

Despite some direct exchanges, the connections interviewees made with other queer women on Instagram tended to be brief and fairly vague. While Mita provided advice through direct messages, she was annoyed when other users wanted to have ongoing conversations over days or months. These connections did not translate into friendships or close relationships because Instagram exchanges did not spark opportunities for deeper, regular bonding time, and Mita noted that she would rather go for coffee with transwomen she met in her community. Alex, who was in contact with many fans of the androgynous clothing account, noted that flirting rarely held the promise of starting a relationship: "It's just commonplace [on] Instagram, for there to be brief flirtations and short friendships and then it's kind of a revolving door: more people coming in, other people kind of slipping out." Among the volume of users and content flows, the possibility for reaching out only led to brief encounters.

Participants frequently felt a sense of connection with other queer women merely through the act of viewing their content or following accounts. Although Julie was not comfortable using queer women's hashtags, making sure to obscure the salience of her sexual identity due to her line of work in Christian-based children's programming, she followed many LGBTQ users under the assumption that her homophobic and religious audiences would not pay close attention to her follower list. She stressed that LGBTQ content was a motivator for using the platform: "I feel connected just through looking even though I don't actually hashtag LGBT." Similarly, as part of the viewership for queer female YouTubers and celebrities, Thea followed these personalities on Instagram because it "makes me feel more included in the community. . . . A lot of them just post like, everyday pictures of what they're doing and stuff, so it makes you feel like maybe you're actually friends with them or, you know, you have more insight into their lives." She invoked the term "community" despite never conversing with any of these individuals.

These loose affinities resonate with Berlant's (2008) description of intimate publics as conveying a sense of community that is undefined. They note, "the feeling of rich continuity with a vaguely defined set of like others is often the central affective magnet of an intimate public" (p. 7). These women were affectively captured by the queer, female identities they saw displayed through hashtags and were often motivated to contribute their own content as a result. But their connections were ultimately vague—made up of an identification of likeness and short exchanges of affirmation. This vagueness, however, sustained the promise of the intimate public as presenting possible images of the good life and brighter futures, since specificity threatens to preclude individuals from seeing themselves in such fantasies.

Instagram's affordances and dominant platform practices—its platform vernacular (Meese et al., 2015)—contributed to a moderate level of salience in queer women's sexual identity expressions, which shaped this loosely connected public. With the platform's array of filters and common practices of glamorous self-display, sexual identity was often portrayed in images on queer women's hashtags as a stylistic feature or brand aesthetic. These images showed how to live, and sometimes how to thrive, within a dominant heteronormative consumer culture, but they rarely challenged it. These portrayals reflect Berlant's (2008) observation that intimate publics are "juxtapolitical," or near politics but necessarily separate from them, serving to give "relief from the political" (p. 10). By widely circulating nonheterosexual female identities, this queer women's intimate public on Instagram was nearly political. But it simultaneously refrained from politics in circulating homonormative fantasies and consumer lifestyles that flourish in ways complicit with—or in spite of—current political conditions rather than fighting them.

This is not to say that such an intimate public does not serve a purpose. In Olszanowski's (2015) study of a networked intimate public of female artists on Instagram, she found that these artists initiated meaningful connections through their shared art practices, focus on displaying the female body, and shared risk of censorship by Instagram and the wider world. Intimate publics, including those restructured through networked platforms, provide centralized representation for marginalized identities and an affective outlet that can be necessary not only for survival but also for looking toward the future. Instagram's intimate public of queer women circulated images of what a desirable, successful individual's life could look like (potentially, when she grows up) even if nothing changes.

VINE'S SOCIABLE COUNTERPUBLICS

In contrast to soft and subtle Instagram imagery, Vines filled up the senses. Across hashtags like #LGBTCrew and #RainbowGang, queer women's spontaneous, often loud, and minimally edited content dominated. While gender-specific hashtags like #lesbehonest or #girlswholikegirls sometimes appeared alongside these tags, they were less popular and appeared to be less necessary, given the large volume of queer women's Vines that overwhelmed broader hashtags. Many of these 6.5-second videos constituted quick check-ins, greetings to an assumed audience, and mundane clips, such as a shot of the view while walking. In her YouTube research, Patricia Lange (2009) developed the term "videos of affinity" for content aiming to build and maintain connections with others. Videos of affinity are often informal and unprompted, and convey in-jokes or personal glimpses of life while making references that resonate with a target audience. They also incorporate the body as a mechanism for fostering affinity. Queer female Viners generated this closeness through videos captured in the personal spaces of their bedrooms, bathrooms, and cars. They held the phone physically close, filming with the front-facing camera to give a sense of proximity and realness through bumps and shakes occurring in the absence of a tripod. A Vine's 6.5 seconds were often consumed by a particular look into the camera, a sigh, or an expression of emotion that provided a quick glimpse of everyday life—often featuring pets. These videos reflect social media's "phatic culture" (Miller, 2008) through the use of phatic communication, comprised of gestures that do not intrinsically convey information but give off social cues to strengthen relationships. The ease of capturing Vines, alongside a reduced imperative for editing due to a lack of tools and a sea of content, was conducive to circulating affinity-building Vines with phatic expressions among queer women.

Beyond serving as check-ins with one's audience, these videos of affinity often included jokes and experiences that made sexual identity and its intersection with other elements of identity highly salient. Several Vines rapidly divulged stories about relationships. For example, one user's video about issues she had with her ex-girlfriend included the hashtag #TheStrugglesofALesbian, assuming that others who identify as lesbian have had similar experiences. As mentioned in chapter 3, many of Chrissy's videos aimed to be relatable in these ways. Her videos spanned topics well beyond her painting and craftwork, and she discussed her motivation to share Vines that displayed multiple facets of her identity: "I feel like I'm stuck in the middle, being in the LGBT community, because it's hard to be a lesbian and be pro-Black without conviction. It's hard to be a lesbian mom without conviction. It's hard to be . . . lesbian and married and pro-Black all at the same time." Her conviction translated into an unabashed display of her sexual identity, Black identity, and role as a wife and mother in clips featuring daily life along with skits and jokes.

Chrissy also participated on LGBTQ and Black Viner hashtags, sometimes together and at other times separately. For example, contributing to the remixes of @Dom's viral "Do it for the Vine" video,[2] Chrissy replicated its rhythm and format in a skit where she played both a mother, telling her child to do her chores, and a defiant child saying, "I ain't gonna do it." Scenes flicked between the two characters until the mother threatened, "[I'll] whoop your ass!" and the child responded, "I'mma do it!" Chrissy posted the Vine with the hashtag #blackmothers, tying into what she views as a relatable experience among fellow Black Viners of having a strong, authoritative mother. The skit reflected elements of Black humor that linguist Kendra Calhoun (2019) notes contributed to a dominant form of racial humor on the platform as "the practice of engaging with racial ideologies and race-based experiences" (p. 30). Chrissy's humor and her playfulness with the original Vine's rhythm and wording also connected with the practice of hashtag signifyin' (Brock, 2012; Florini, 2014), building on its responsive, short, networked form of dialogue while integrating Vine's audiovisual affordances. Through self-representations that invited others to connect intimately, relate, and build upon such expressions, queer women participated in the collective building of shared identities on Vine.

Affinity through Sexual Desire

Sexual expression was also key to communicating and connecting through a shared, salient sexual identity. Vine's departure from the static Instagram photo or the silent GIF enabled users to include dynamic movement and sound in videos, adding music to the background long before the platform incorporated tools for doing so. Dance and lip-sync videos abounded, with Vines popularizing dance moves like "the dab" and boosting the fanbase for several hip-hop and pop artists (Josephs, 2016). Many queer women's videos combined lip-syncing and dancing with sensual moves, tight or minimal clothing, and sexual gestures. The videos' sexual nature was often made explicit in captions through flirtatious phrases and emoji, such as

🐱👅💧 (a tongue next to a cat with heart eyes and water droplets) to indicate a desire to perform cunnilingus. Vine's loop allowed sensuality to build over the course of these videos, and users often included the most intensely sexual gestures at the end, inciting viewers to watch again.

These Vines can be linked to a broader social media practice known colloquially as "thirst trapping"—the posting of selfies or self-representations with the intention to "trap" or capture the sexual attention of one's audience. Queer women often made this link explicit through the addition of #ttsquad (short for "thirst trap squad") alongside LGBTQ hashtags on their videos. Thirst, in these cases, refers to the visual enticement of desire, which is deployed with the expectation of a positive response and possible reciprocity (Merriam-Webster, n.d.). While thirst trap videos were popular across Vine, Black queer female Viners were prominent creators of this content. They often danced to rap or hip-hop, frequently including songs from the trap subgenre, which originated in Black communities of the southern United States (Lee, 2015). For example, in 2015, American rapper Willie Junior Maxwell II—known popularly as Fetty Wap—was rising to fame following the release of his hit "Trap Queen" in the previous year. Vine arguably contributed to this listenership, with users including the song in a range of less and more sexual videos (Madden, 2015), including thirst traps. Although many users adopted this genre of music in their videos, Black queer women's thirst traps—especially when posted with LGBTQ and Black Vine hashtags—had the potential to reflect both racial and sexual identity associations.

While dominant platform practices often permeate smaller publics, thirst trapping convened attention around LGBTQ hashtags for fun and flirtatiousness in ways particular to queer female Viners. The songs used in thirst traps were often sung by male musicians and incorporated for their sexually explicit lyrics. As women sang along with or lip-synced this music, their participation could be viewed as taking on a male role in order to express sexual assertiveness. But understanding their Vines in this way reinforces dominant discourses that heterosexualize queer women's sexuality and reify binary gender roles in relationships and sexual encounters (de Lauretis, 1993; Jackson & Gilbertson, 2009). It also misses a key aspect of these performances. I observed female Viners featuring lyrics about giving women sexual pleasure, often cutting off musical segments before misogynistic or degrading portions of songs played. They queerly appropriated these otherwise heteronormative and masculinist songs for female sexual desire. This focus on women in their thirst traps was heightened through the inclusion of queer fashion, unambiguous captions, hashtags, and sexual gestures.

Beyond flirtatiousness, these displays also playfully established and re-inforced social connections. Women made response videos for each other as gifts, such as one thirst trap video posted with a "happy birthday" message for another user. Gender and cultural studies scholar Kane Race (2015) highlights gay men's use of digital technologies to establish "spaces of sexual sociability and redistributions of intimacy" (p. 506). Sexual socia-bility comprises sexual exchanges as well as friendly activities with sexual undertones, such as chatting, watching pornography together, and co-browsing profiles on hook-up apps, giving rise to intimate communities and connections among gay men. While queer women's sexual desire is so often overlooked, their exchanges on Vine reflected a similar sexual socia-bility, spurring these women to connect, produce content for each other, and hold meaningful dialogues. Thirst traps constituted highly salient self-representations of sexual identity that brought women close together, serving the counterpublic purposes of regroupment and building solidarity.

Collective Counterpublic Discourse

Affinity and solidarity among queer female Viners made way for displays of counterpublic discourse. This took place in two overlapping forms: sus-tained dialogue among a counterpublic of LGBTQ users, which garnered sufficient participation to be noticeable and potentially disruptive to the wider platform, and widely circulated and affectively powerful statements challenging dominant discourses. While these forms were evident across my observations of LGBTQ hashtags, interviewees provided vivid descriptions. Chrissy became increasingly involved in a dialogue sus-tained through #nightspeak, a hashtag that represented a user community posting discussion topics on a nightly basis that were "tailored to lesbians." Activity on #nightspeak had a temporal dimension, with the most active users located in the US Eastern Standard time zone kicking off early in the evening, and users across America and internationally joining as the night progressed. Those participating posted a volume of content for each other that, when shared in tandem, resembled a video-based chatroom. Their activity took advantage of the hashtag much in the same way that Twitter users originally imported this practice from Internet Relay Chat, hashtagging to differentiate discussion topics and establish a chat-like structure (Halavais, 2014).

While women on #nightspeak posted about their experiences and perspectives under the shared identity of lesbian, the hashtag's creator steered the conversation. It was common on Vine for originators of popular hashtags to designate themselves as "CEO," often reflected in usernames (if this book had a hashtag, I would be "Stef || CEO #PersonalNotPrivate"). Chrissy told me that #nightspeak's CEO appointed "admins" with whom she communicated behind the scenes via text message to plan topics and ways to sustain the conversation. This added coordination is likely what transformed the gathering of women from a counterpublic of strangers into a sustained community in which individuals became more familiar with each other.

When Chrissy became an admin, she saw firsthand how topics she started could generate such a large volume of content that users outside this community were compelled to take notice, "Everybody—big Viners got on the hashtag, small Viners got on the hashtag, and we trended number one." This high level of activity propelled #nightspeak to the top of Vine's "Trending Tags" section, grabbing the attention of users across the platform. Similarly, the tendency for hashtags associated with Black Twitter to trend, due to their high level of dialogic participation, was one of the ways they garnered attention from the rest of that platform (Brock, 2012). The ability to circulate topics through a lesbian-oriented hashtag and into the view of others across Vine constituted a powerful form of counterpublic disruption that #nightspeak participants wielded to draw attention to their lives and experiences.

While these hashtag-specific conversations occurred according to temporal rhythms, several users posted videos to broader LGBTQ hashtags to make statements or get across messages challenging heterosexism, ignorance, or intersectional forms of discrimination. Narrative skits were a popular form of humor across the platform, with users frequently adding depth to this genre of one-person acting through the use of props or costumes to construct multiple characters—reflected in Chrissy's chore skit—contributing to "instant characterization" (Marone, 2017, p. 55) communicated expediently across short scenes. With her improvisation training, Jaxx was talented at transforming real-life scenarios of homophobia, ableism, and ethnic stereotyping into skits that called out this behavior. One of her Vines commenced with an imposing close-up as a distressed character who states, "You're going to hell!" Jaxx hears this response frequently when disclosing her sexual identity. She followed it with a scene as herself, wiping away fake tears with a rainbow flag, sarcastically wondering, "Oh no, whatever will I do? I will be going to a place surrounded by other lesbians who are horny and willing."

Jaxx described these skits as "a way to bounce back at people who are ignorant." She was astounded by their positive reception when cross-posted to Tumblr, which has historically been a refuge for LGBTQ youth to make discoveries about their sexual and gender identities through its queer archive of content and affordances for connecting with like-minded others (Cho, 2015; Robards et al., 2018). Jaxx's fans saw their experiences represented in her skits and also shared them widely to further her challenge to oppressive and normative discourses. She was moved by messages from her Tumblr followers, especially an email from a young woman outside the United States: "She lives in a country where she would be killed if she was out. . . . She started talking about how my Vine—she's like, it makes her happy to know there are people like me that are able to speak out for a community and live my life and be happy and proud in a way that she can't be. And that watching my Vines just filled her with joy, and I'm like, 'My dumb Vines?' And then I'm like, 'Wow, my dumb Vines.'"

Humor, especially the online variety, is often dismissed in this way as "dumb," frivolous, or an otherwise vapid pastime. However, Jaxx's videos were propelled into a range of publics where users might post them as a form of entertainment as well as a means of collective identification, a mechanism of confrontation, or an invocation for others to challenge intolerant behavior and attitudes. They represent a broadening of the antihegemonic racial humor that Calhoun (2019) found on Vine, which aimed to critique, contradict, and complicate racial stereotypes while providing alternative narratives. Building on these user practices and emergent genres of Vine humor, LGBTQ users applied such techniques ·to matters of sexual and gender identity. Their circulation of such counterdiscourses reflects the efforts of counterpublics to realize a different world through forms of address that challenge the status quo (Warner, 2002).

RENDERING SALIENCE TARGETABLE

Platforms certainly played a role in the kinds of queer women's publics that formed on Instagram and Vine as well as the salience with which sexual identity could be expressed, given that representations of sexual identity and sexuality often incurred negative repercussions. Platforms' technical infrastructures and governance approaches contributed to circumstances in which queer women's salient representations of sexual identity were targeted for censorship, harassment, or discrimination. Instagram's stringent policies against nudity, co-moderation system that encourages users to police each other, and banning of certain hashtags all worked to constrain the reach of queer women's content. In contrast, Vine's relaxed policies and circulation of racist and misogynist content paved the way for a barrage of hateful comments and harassment targeting those who spoke out against it.

In the Platform's Crosshairs

Instagram's policies prohibit users from posting nudity, with some exceptions for works of art and—more recently—photos of breastfeeding and mastectomy scars, following campaigns demanding the platform #freethenipple (West, 2017). Olszanowski (2014) observes that these policies are communicated in ways that are pejorative and shaming toward bodies and acts that involve nudity, with Instagram's community guidelines quipping, "Keep your clothes on" (p. 87). The guidelines also incite users to police each other to "help us keep the community strong" (Instagram, 2015, 2020). This is supported through flagging functionality within the platform, which allows users to report others' content for removal. This sort of co-moderation, in which responsibility is distributed among users and the platform, is a common governance approach, in part due to the large scale of activity to which these companies must attend. But flagging systems often obscure the platform's role in moderation and make it appear neutral (Crawford & Gillespie, 2016). By framing nudity as shameful and asking others to get involved when they see this content, Instagram is anything but neutral in handing over the reins of moderation to its users and providing little recourse for those who are flagged.

An incident with Alex's androgynous clothing account on Instagram is a prime example of how platform co-moderation can lead to individuals being targeted even when they do not violate Instagram's policies. Alex commissioned a professional photoshoot with models showcasing the underwear line. One image became wildly popular on Instagram: it depicted a woman in a black bra and panties poised over another woman in a denim vest who was wearing the briefs Alex had designed. Both women's genitals and nipples were covered and their bodies were not touching, as the shot captured the more femininely dressed woman leaning in for a kiss. While other fashion accounts, such as Victoria's Secret with its lingerie models, commonly revealed as much or more skin, this did not prevent Alex's photo from being flagged. In contrast to Alex's models, who displayed same-gender attraction along with gender nonconforming fashion and visible tattoos, Victoria's Secret models adhere to normative standards of beauty and femininity, which seem to make them less of a target for moderation.

"It was a warning," Alex recalled about the notification from Instagram. "They were saying my account could be deleted." Having expended time and effort building a following, Alex opted to remove the photo rather than challenge Instagram, acknowledging that the account was more vulnerable than others to these sorts of censorship: "You see girls all the time in less, but I think there are a lot of really homophobic people that like to just bash on, um, my page and I think it was probably one of them." Instagram's ban on nudity, paired with the ability of any homophobic or heterosexist user to flag an image and invoke swift action regardless of whether it actually violates the policy, made this an expected occurrence.

Why would Instagram be so reactive without verifying that the flagging and censorship of queer women's bodies at least accords with their policies? Aside from the additional time and money required for human moderators to evaluate content, my research indicated that queer women's images were caught up in another issue that Instagram attempted to solve through highly responsive takedowns. As I queried Instagram's application programming interface (API)[3] for images posted to queer women's hashtags, the program I used returned results starting with those most recently posted. This unearthed many commercial pornographic images and videos, indicating that Instagram deals with a barrage of pornography second by second. Most users are likely in the dark about this issue, as much of this content was removed in a matter of minutes when I searched for it through Instagram's user interface. Even so, several women I interviewed noted pornographic content on the hashtags they perused. Julie exclaimed, "Especially if I click the word 'lesbian,' next thing you know, it becomes a big porn festival and that's not at all what I was having in mind." While these women were not averse to sexual content, they observed sexist and heteronormative themes across these images. Queenie articulated the difference: "It's the wider idea of lesbians in porn, you know, it's not really healthy, safe, GLBT porn. It's the traditional, fake everything, not real at all." Participants recounted images that perpetuated the common heterosexual pornographic trope of "lesbians" as women engaged in same-gender sexual activity for men's pleasure (Jenefsky & Miller, 1998). These posts often attempted to draw users to paid pornography websites or instant messaging apps (e.g., Kik or Snapchat), reflecting the capacity of pornography to double as spam. As such, Instagram's moderation efforts ramped up on these hashtags to target content that violated both its policies on nudity and repetitive commercial solicitation.

This intensive moderation of queer women's hashtags contributes to further censorship of their content. When hashtags become associated with a large amount of content in violation of platform policies, Instagram "bans" them, effectively rendering their content invisible in searches. While users can still add banned hashtags to their posts, hashtag searches return only select "top posts" or no results even if the search bar indicates that thousands of images with this hashtag exist. For example, a search for #lesbian in 2017 indicated that it was used in 3,309,460 posts, but only a handful of images appeared at the top of the search page. These were followed by a notice that read: "Recent posts from #lesbian are currently hidden because the community has reported some content that may not meet Instagram's community guidelines." Pointing to "the community" as the cause for this censorship obscures whether the reported content was commercial spam or queer women's photos abiding by the nudity policy. It also erases the role of automated systems and algorithmic content moderation, associating removal specifically with humans as community members.

Scholars have identified that algorithmic pornography filters are disproportionately trained to recognize feminine figures (Gehl et al., 2017), and it may only be a matter of time before Instagram follows in Facebook's footsteps to employ algorithmic moderation systems for nudity (Gorwa et al., 2020). Law scholars Alice Witt, Nicolas Suzor, and Anna Huggins (2019) argue that within Instagram's opaque moderation processes "the lack of formal equality, certainty, reason giving and user participation, and Instagram's largely unfettered power to moderate content with limited transparency and accountability, are significant normative concerns which pose an ongoing risk of arbitrariness for women and users more broadly" (p. 562). Arbitrariness was exactly what concerned the queer women I interviewed. Queenie reflected, "For some reason [pornographic images] get by somehow while other artistic photos or even some photos promoting breast cancer awareness and things like that, they get flagged and taken down." As a burlesque dancer, plus-size model, and activist, she was never sure when her content would be subject to flagging and removal. Overall, Instagram's stringent policies, co-moderation, and active censorship can be understood as contributing to the vague, commercial, and sterile nature of the intimate networked public among queer women on the platform.

Users Taking Aim

While takedowns like the one Alex experienced indicate that some individuals targeted queer women through formal moderation procedures, users on both platforms also subjected the women I spoke with to more direct forms of discriminatory, harassing, and sexualized content. Following from Twitter's history of relatively relaxed terms of service in comparison to Facebook and Instagram (Curtis, 2019), Vine was also less stringent than Instagram regarding content moderation. On the one hand, this enabled sexual sociability and counterpublic discourse among queer women. Vine's accommodation of "suggestive posts, just not sexually explicit ones" in its "Explicit Sexual Policy" protected flirtatious thirst traps with a specific caveat exempting videos with "clothed sexually suggestive dancing" from removal. On the other hand, Vine's "Sensitive Media" policy allowed hateful content to remain on the platform. It stated that videos containing "disparaging speech regarding others based on race, religious affiliation, national origin, ethnicity, gender, gender identity, sexual orientation, serious disease, or disability" could be marked as "sensitive and potentially a violation of the Vine Rules." Videos marked as "sensitive" required users to click/tap to view them instead of autoplaying in feeds. This policy positioned Vine as the discerning power designating videos as "sensitive," providing a mechanism for such content to remain on the platform and leaving room for discriminatory content to thrive through the blurry language of "potential" violation.

Although it is unclear how often videos were designated as "sensitive," Chrissy and Jaxx spoke of regularly encountering sexist, homophobic, and misogynistic content. Often these videos appeared without the "sensitive" filter, allowing them to autoplay and gain the momentum to appear in top-ranked sections of the app. Jaxx recalled encounters with "racist humor and there's a lot of like, 'my side chick' and all that kind of fuckboy humor on Vine." With humor as a trending genre, Viners' videos discussing cheating on their girlfriends (with a "side chick") and racist jokes were prominent. "Fuckboy" has emerged in popular culture as an identifier for men who sexually objectify women or spread misogynistic views (Boboltz, 2015). Jaxx asserted that Vine's most prominent and popular content reflected its status as "Straight White Boy Fuckboy Central," with these users' content setting the platform's tone. Communication scholar Adrienne Massanari's (2015) research addresses similar waves of sexist and misogynistic content on Reddit. Her concept of "toxic technocultures" describes "toxic cultures that are enabled by and propagated through sociotechnical networks," characterized by "an Othering of those perceived as outside the culture" (p. 333). Toxic cultures leverage platform affordances to reinforce and circulate harmful attitudes, building divides of inclusion and exclusion often defined by lines of gender, sexual identity, and race. Such a combination gives rise to technocultural practices that target excluded others to the point of affecting their ability to use the platform as well as threatening them in mentally and physically damaging ways (e.g., "doxxing" by revealing one's legal name and/or physical location so they can be stalked or harassed in person). The ability for racist, sexist, and homophobic Viners to circulate their content widely generated and reinforced a toxic technoculture that actively targeted women, people of color, and queer people.

Vine's toxic technoculture manifested through consistent harassment as waves of negative, insulting, threatening, and discriminatory messages and comments on queer women's videos. Chrissy referred to this collectively as "The Hate" and noted that she was targeted for both her racial and sexual identity: "I got so much hate when I first started Vine because I was a lesbian and I was Black." She recounted a particularly jarring incident: "I had this white guy tell me, 'You're like the worst combination in life because you're—not only are you homosexual but you're Black." These comments went far beyond critiquing her content and attacked her identity in ways that were hurtful but were only a "potential" violation of Vine's policies.

Jaxx spoke about the bittersweet experience of having a video featured in Vine's comedy section, where it gained attention that could propel her popularity: "It's a double-edged sword because part of you is like, 'Great, awesome!' in being on the Comedy page. And part of you is like, 'Here comes the wave of fuckboys.'" Jaxx's description of a "wave" and Chrissy's reference to "The Hate" indicate that this volume of harassment is experienced as an overwhelming barrage—a force intrinsic to both the platform and its dominant user culture. Jaxx felt this backlash spoke to the impact of queer, racialized women's videos: "White boys get angry when women start to talk about their life experiences, especially if [the women] are gay." Life narratives that convened counterpublics relating to sexual identity, race, and other marginal identities were threatening to those who derived power from oppressing these populations. Media scholar Sarah Banet-Weiser (2018) identifies this ebb and flow between highly visible feminist expression and misogynistic responses. She explains, "The restoration of male privilege is the logical crux of the mirroring effect I see between popular feminism and popular misogyny" (p. 38). Through misogynistic responses, some men seek to regain their power within patriarchal systems that often disenfranchise women and render them invisible in public space. Banet-Weiser underscores digital media's focal role in the circulation of discourses pertaining to both popular feminism and popular misogyny. However, Vine offered little recourse against reactive waves of misogyny, with the act of blocking harassers requiring dedicated time and emotional labor, only to have them reappear through new pseudonymous accounts.

Instagram was not devoid of this behavior, but harassment often took the form of sexual aggression, which sought to reassert the dominance of heterosexuality and punish homosexual expression. Queenie, whose burlesque photoshoots attracted a great deal of attention from men, noticed a surge in hostile comments when she posted photos with her gender nonconforming partner. She explained, "I think for some of the straight male followers that I had, who would comment or like the photos that I had that were scantily clad or things like that, I think knowing I was a lesbian was a turn-off for them because they couldn't imagine things, to be honest." Given that Instagram already calls on users to police each other's sexual expression, it comes as no surprise that users feel comfortable criticizing relationships that do not align with heterosexualizing fantasies of lesbian relationships.

Women on both platforms regularly received direct messages containing nonconsensual sexually explicit material. This made inboxes unusable for connecting with strangers, with Chrissy noting that she did not check messages outside of her "friends" filter "because we get a lot of nasty Vines that are, like, genitals." Instagram's stringent policy against nudity did not prevent users from receiving sexually suggestive imagery from men. Mïta capitalized the words "LESBIAN" and "MARRIED" in her profile due to the onslaught of unsolicited explicit photos users sent by direct message: "What I was getting with Kik and I still get with Instagram—though not as much—is the fucking dick pics. I just—it makes me throw up, right? Like, I don't want to see that stuff. What goes through a person's mind that makes—like that tells them 'yes, this is a good decision?'" Several studies reveal that the photos men send nonconsensually to women of their genitalia—"dick pics"—are often viewed more widely by authorities and institutions as a joke and rarely incur negative consequences (Albury, 2015; Dobson, 2015). This allows men on social media to send dick pics with little worry about repercussions. However, nonconsensual and sexually aggressive messages can be understood as assertions of masculine dominance over women (Hess & Flores, 2018). In the case of queer women frequently receiving dick pics, these images may also attempt to reinforce the dominance of heterosexuality, reflecting the violent perspective that lesbians can be *turned straight* through a sexual encounter with a man. Transgender women also experience sexual fetishization from cisgender men (Gercio, 2015). In these ways, the harassing content that queer women must deflect in their everyday use of these platforms reflects not only the rampant sexualization of women online but also the policing and punishment of queer sexual identities.

CONCLUSION: NOWHERE TO GO UNDER PATCHWORK PLATFORM GOVERNANCE

This chapter has shown how collective identity signaling on contemporary platforms can give rise to publics and counterpublics. Individuals' engagement with platforms in processes of identity modulation can enhance the salience of their sexual identity in self-representations, generating the texts around which users gather as publics. Salience makes people highly recognizable, even relatable, to each other. On Instagram, the salience of others' sexual identities contributed to a vague sense of community, in which some queer women found motivation and affirmation. The lesbian digital dreamgirl, as a highly salient representation circulated through queer women's hashtags, provides a model for economic success and ideal citizenship within neoliberal logics. In contrast, counterpublics convened on Vine through videos displaying personal elements of affinity, sexual sociability, and strong counternormative discourses challenged existing logics and biases. Through videos that critiqued intersecting inequalities relating to sexual identity as well as race and ability, queer women engaged in counterpublic "world making" (Warner, 2002), wielding salient representations of identity to carve out space for a world where they would be able to thrive. Platforms contributed to these modes of identity modulation, with Instagram's platform vernacular of luxury and consumption rewarding apolitical representations, and Vine's affective looping functionality and relaxed policies allowing for highly personal sexual expression and impactful narratives.

However, platforms' governance policies and their technological scaffolding also place limitations on the salience of queer women's self-representations. Jean Burgess, Nicolas Suzor, and I (Duguay et al., 2018) have argued that this is an implication of patchwork platform governance, an approach to governing users that focuses "on formal policies and procedures of content moderation while failing to address substantive cultures of use and the technological mechanisms that sustain them" (p. 240). These kinds of governance measures are often developed retroactively once an issue has become highly visible in the media or if pressure is placed on a platform to change its policy, as in the case of Instagram eventually permitting breastfeeding photos. Formal policies, when paired with co-moderation mechanisms of flagging content and blocking users, can make queer women targets of censorship either through overregulation that still fails to curb commercial (pornographic) spam or at the whim of homophobic users.

Often governance policies mix with platforms' profit motives and aim to appeal to advertisers, such as the changes YouTube made to its advertising structure in 2017. Purportedly in efforts to curb extremist content, these changes rendered LGBTQ users' content unavailable in "Restricted Mode," a setting intended to restrict mature content, such as profanity and violence. Restricted mode reduced these creators' search visibility and demonetized their videos by removing pre-roll advertisements even when their content was not mature but simply discussed LGBTQ-related matters (Southerton et al., 2021). Such policies and their enforcement mechanisms make platforms appear responsive to advertiser concerns about their brands being shown in conjunction with controversial content, while LGBTQ users serve as collateral damage in profit-generation strategies.

Platforms' moderation features are also insufficient to protect queer women from becoming targets of large-scale harassment and discrimination. Patchwork platform governance specifically overlooks toxic technocultures, as policies and moderation mechanisms pose few consequences for misogynistic, heterosexist, and racist behavior. Several scholars echo this chapter's findings that platforms' algorithms and ranking functionalities are often complicit in the circulation of discriminatory content and can reward its originators with increased visibility (see, e.g., Matamoros-Fernández, 2017; Noble, 2018). Patchwork platform governance places queer women in the crosshairs of platform censorship and user harassment, leading them to self-censor, participate less, and sometimes reach a breaking point of leaving a platform altogether. Porting content and followers elsewhere is difficult, so these barriers to participation decimate counterpublics while platforms effectively protect and continue to profit from those who perpetuate toxic technocultures.

Several women I spoke with mentioned Tumblr as a refuge from platform censorship and relentless harassment. Indeed, scholars have pointed to Tumblr as a home for queer youth in their identity development (Wargo, 2015), transgender community building (Fink & Miller, 2014; Haimson et al., 2019), women sharing "not safe for work" (NSFW) images that defy body normativity (Tiidenberg & Gomez Cruz, 2015), and queer expression more broadly.[4] In his study of an asexual counterpublic on Tumblr, Renninger (2015) identifies that the platform differs from Facebook and Instagram through features and practices that afford counterpublic communication. Among these are the use of pseudonyms and content-sharing conventions that involve "reblogging," posting something to one's blog to share it, which effectively holds users accountable for the content they circulate.

In addition to these affordances, Tumblr allowed for the sharing of NSFW content, though it was filtered in different ways over time, sometimes complicating access to it (Gillespie, 2013). Anthropologist Alexander Cho (2015) observes how this erotic content flowed among queer Tumblr users along with pictures of art, landscapes, and GIFs from pop culture. He describes the affective intensity as well as the ebbs and flows of this content as a form of queer "reverb," also drawing on notions of sound. Reverb occurs through repetition and endures over time. He explains, "Reverb is a quality and a process, a way to understand the direction and intensity of the flows of affect" (p. 53). Within a framework of identity modulation, the affective intensity of intimate, sexual, emotional queer content shared to Tumblr could be thought of as comprising highly salient representations of sexual identity, which reverberated through Tumblr's affordances as it was repeatedly encountered, shared, and sustained through flows of circulation.

But everything changed in December 2018. Tumblr's CEO Jeff D'Onofrio (2018) posted an announcement that the platform would no longer allow adult content. This decision followed Verizon's acquisition of Yahoo! (Tumblr's parent company) in 2017 and occurred amid controversy linked to allegations of hosting child pornography, which led app stores to temporarily ban the app (Tiidenberg, Hendry, & Abidin, 2021). Tumblr's updated policy banned depictions of sex, genitals, and "female-presenting nipples," a term garnering criticism for its gender essentialism. While Tumblr asserted that these changes would reinforce the platform as a safe space for developing a sense of community, media scholar Paul Byron's (2019) analysis of user reactions indicates that is exactly what was lost. He writes that users' outcry speaks to "how feelings of safety, freedom, and creativity require space that is open to many uses and many bodies, rather than a space guided by overarching rules that determine sexual content as 'violation'" (p. 13). While adult content was not all that sustained Tumblr's queer communities, it contributed to an intimacy and affective intensity conducive to identity development and the formation of networked counterpublics. Its ban tells these users that their bodies, desires, affects, and counterdiscourses no longer belong on a platform prioritizing commercial viability as Tumblr falls in line with Facebook and Instagram in the broader sterilization of popular platforms.

Shortly after the news broke about Tumblr, CBC (2019) interviewed Cho and I separately for a radio segment. When asked, "How do you think LGBTQ youth will respond to these new changes on Tumblr?" I reflected on the massive number of posts from users threatening to leave the platform and shared my belief that some youth would turn to lesser-known platforms. They may migrate to Mastodon, I suggested, a decentralized networking service hosted on different servers, which gives communities the agency to choose specific terms of service rather than one set of rules enforced across communities. However, I raised issues with this: such a migration to gated communities loses the heterogeneity of popular platforms and potential of forming publics and counterpublics among many different people uniting over shared elements of identity. It also raises the bar for digital literacy and the need for individuals to conform to identity markers of more homogenous communities, such as the lesbian signifiers required by members of the Sappho listserv.

With a 30 percent decline in web traffic months after Tumblr's ban on adult content (Liao, 2019), some users certainly jumped ship. But Cho predicted that many LGBTQ youth would stay: "I saw someone posting about how there really were no alternative spaces and that they really didn't want to switch to Twitter because, in their words, 'Twitter was heterosexual Tumblr with less options and more obnoxious trolls.'" He conjectured that although Tumblr content would become less edgy, queer young people had built communities for which other platforms provided lesser affordances. Further, platform policies were becoming uniform in ways that left youth with little choice for outlets allowing for more sexual expression and the same quality of dialogue. He concluded, "I'm not sure where else these queer kids are going to be able to go." Indeed, a quick search of Tumblr hashtags reveals that it is still full of (now sanitized) LGBTQ content.

In a way, Cho and I raised similar concerns. Publics are powerful in their ability to convene strangers around a shared text (Warner, 2002): a shared focus of attention, affect, intimacy, and identity. The patchwork platform governance of popular platforms and their persistence in moderating, regulating, and eradicating sexual content means that there remain few spaces where queer people can encounter a diversity of strangers with whom to form publics and counterpublics. Lesser-known platforms afford gated communities, which can be important for the regroupment of counterpublics. However, they do not allow the same circulation of counterpublic discourse, which platforms like Tumblr and Vine previously did, enabling posts to be amplified to those who may not otherwise encounter messages against homophobia, misogyny, and racism. As the fate of these platforms shows, while these technologies hold much possibility for identity modulation to contribute to impactful forms of collective representation, their decommissioning or adoption of uniform policies is leaving us with nowhere to go with our world-making statements of identity.

CHAPTER 5

Conclusion

Identity Modulation as Integral to Digital Citizenship

In making sense of this research in a broader context of negotiating identity and personal disclosure on social media, I have become aware of just how often circumstances repeat. Initially drafting this conclusion midway through 2020, working from home during the novel coronavirus (COVID-19) pandemic, life is on a loop: news websites refresh to show higher case numbers by the hour, cities ease restrictions then return to lockdown after new outbreaks, the latest season of *Queer Eye* plays in the background, and I swear I've seen this makeover before. TikTok has become part of the repetitious din filling pandemic time, as the app's uptake soared in early 2020 (Pham, 2020). With similarities to Vine, TikTok allows users to share short looping clips, trending strongly toward dance and lip-sync videos queued to music, fueled by the app's 2018 merger with Musical.ly (Mercuri, 2018). I downloaded it tentatively, not certain whether its looping media would help to pass time or make it stand still, but feeling obliged when I heard that queer content abounded across users' videos.

In June 2020, the *New York Times* (NYT) ran a story by columnist Lena Wilson (2020) entitled, "For Lesbians, TikTok Is 'The Next Tinder,'" which featured women who met on the app and started relationships. The article links to a post in which Lauren Vlach, a user with more than forty-five thousand followers at the time, records a date with her girlfriend, whom she met on the app, with a caption claiming this, "proves Tik Tok [*sic*] is the best lesbian dating app." Wilson proceeds to discuss "Lesbian TikTok" as a "corner of

Personal but Not Private. Stefanie Duguay, Oxford University Press. © Oxford University Press 2022.
DOI: 10.1093/oso/9780190076184.003.0005

the app" dominated by lesbian references that facilitate a sense of community. For example, with TikTok's prominent music integration, responding "Yes" to "Do you listen to Girl in Red?"[1]—a queer musician—has become short-hand for coming out. This practice resembles Phyllis's line of questioning for Tinder users about Kristen Stewart's sexuality, mentioned in chapter 2, as a way to gauge identity through shared cultural literacy.[2] Queer women on TikTok also engage in technocultural practices resulting in identity-related expressions similar to those chronicled in this book. For example, drawing on the platform's audiovisual affordances, some showcase "cottagecore" imagery of immersive nature scenes with nostalgic undertones of lesbian homesteading culture (Slone, 2020). In these instances, music, hashtags, and looping functionality come together with historical and contemporary references to lesbian culture. Wilson situates Lesbian TikTok within the context of digital technologies, and the internet in general, as providing means for LGBTQ people to connect, especially for youth who have not yet come out, and lauds TikTok as "a place where they can do so safely."

But TikTok is a more complicated platform for queer self-representation than the article lets on. The Chinese technology company ByteDance owns TikTok and a similar app specific to China's technology market, Douyin. Scholars observe that Douyin and TikTok function in parallel, but Douyin has been complicit in serving the Chinese state's political goals, such as by showcasing #PositiveEnergy videos with patriotic discourse (Chen et al., 2020). While the Chinese government decriminalized homosexuality in 1997 and declassified it as a mental disorder in 2001, same-sex marriage remains illegal, and stigma endures against LGBTQ people (Baculinao, 2020; Chen, 2018). In 2018, another popular Chinese platform, Weibo, banned *homosexual content* under a broader initiative also targeting violent and pornographic content in order to make the platform more "harmonious" (Chappell, 2018). Although Weibo quickly reversed this decision in light of public outcry, it serves as an example of how precarious queer representations of identity may be when hosted on platforms with governance models subject to state and cultural ideologies (from which US platforms are not exempt, as this chapter later underscores in discussing Facebook's selective governance decisions).

While several privacy concerns have been raised over TikTok's ownership by a Chinese company (Fowler, 2020), they tend to point more broadly to issues of large-scale data collection and algorithmic processing that occur on many platforms, especially US-based behemoths like Google and Facebook. These concerns align with Cheney-Lippold's (2017) arguments that platforms' datafication of users' personal information is used to generate algorithmic identities that can shape not only individuals' experiences on a platform but also how they are treated as consumers and citizens on-line and offline. TikTok's algorithmic personalization is strong, providing users with highly curated content, to the extent that a woman interviewed in the NYT article revealed that she thought Lesbian TikTok was "the only TikTok" (Wilson, 2020). Following the networked accounts of lesbians and liking content with lesbian-related hashtags populated her feed with more lesbians. The resulting homogeneity of content becomes alarming when considering what gets included or excluded from individuals' feeds. Who makes it into Lesbian TikTok? For whom is this a safe space? And for whom is it a potentially lucrative space? What are users missing when the *safe space* becomes all they see on a platform where so much else is happening?

In 2019, the Intercept obtained documents from TikTok's internal mod-eration guidelines instructing that certain users should not appear in the app's personalized "For You" section based on their appearance (e.g., "ab-normal body shape") or surroundings, such as videos shot in a house with a "slummy character" (Biddle et al., 2020). Responding to criticism that these policies support the suppression of videos by disabled and lower-in-come users, a TikTok representative defended the policies as an attempt to prevent bullying. Other reports noted that TikTok gave this explana-tion to highlight its aim to *protect* people prone to harassment, including LGBTQ people, though the creators subject to these policies did not appre-ciate that protection equated to deplatforming (Botella, 2019). Moreover, the policy documents reveal efforts to generate a particular aesthetic on the platform, avoiding featuring videos depicting environments that are "less fancy and appealing." Examples in previous chapters show that this is not the first time a platform has tried to draw attention to certain users or favor specific practices of self-representation to attain a particular aes-thetic that appeals to mainstream audiences. Although TikTok asserts that this moderation policy has been abandoned, its legacy and the pronounced influence of the app's algorithm on content demonstrates immense inter-vention in users' reach.

Lesbian TikTok is an apt illustration of users producing media that reflects a personal facet of identity—specifically, lesbian identity—in negotiation with app affordances that shape these self-representations and the possibilities that can be realized through them, such as the pos-sibility of meeting one's next girlfriend. Some of these affordances, such as hashtags and looping video, are not new—after all, TikTok was often compared to Vine in its debut (Langford, 2019)—but they are embedded in new arrangements of features; emergent user communities; and broader platform contexts of governance, business models, and so-ciopolitical influences. Through this book's conceptual framework of identity modulation, individuals' agentic personal disclosures have been examined within platform-specific arrangements to identify how personal identifiability, reach, and salience are adjusted—modulated—in apparently seamless negotiations between users and platforms. Although a close analysis of TikTok and investigation into the experiences of its lesbian users would be necessary to understand specific identity modulation processes taking place on this platform, it is already possible from the NYT article to identify how such dynamics may be playing out. Some affordances repeat across platforms, and some cultural references endure over time (I've already spotted many backwards hats on TikTok). Examining these alongside new iterations of technical features and cultural production through the lens of identity modulation makes it possible to see the opportunities these negotiations open up, ranging from one-on-one connections to the formation of world-making publics and counterpublics—a Lesbian TikTok for finding both romance and solace during a global pandemic.

However, identity modulation as a sensitizing framework also makes clear when platform arrangements get in the way of individuals' personal disclosures and self-representations. More than this, it helps to identify when platforms put users at risk of deception, harassment, and homophobia; censor their bodies; and curtail their audiences. Here is where I join the ranks of scholars who repeatedly state that platforms must do more to protect and empower their users. From an initial glance, it appears that platforms have design elements that trip users up, and quick changes can ameliorate these. However, new features and functionalities are insufficient when platforms operate within political, economic, and social realms that have significant impacts on users' well-being and communities. In this final chapter, I highlight some of the hindrances to user agency over identity modulation that this book has uncovered, pointing toward how they can be addressed at multiple levels and, ultimately, by entrenching identity modulation within the suite of rights that comprise digital citizenship. Acting on any of these levels will cut through the repetition in how similar arrangements across platforms inhibit identity modulation, especially in relation to sexuality and sexual identity but also more broadly in the intimate sharing of oneself.

CHALLENGES FOR IDENTITY MODULATION

This book has shown how platforms and individuals mutually contribute to processes of identity modulation, which give rise to digitally mediated representations of identity. Many examples in previous chapters involved hurdles for individuals in disclosing and managing their personal information as well as the audiences who receive it. These hurdles certainly have to do with platform infrastructure, design, features, and functionalities that complicate identity modulation, many of which have been identified by scholars as components of platforms that facilitate context collapse and jeopardize privacy (Cho, 2017; Marwick & boyd, 2014; Zhao et al., 2013). Several queer women I spoke with mentioned platform mechanisms that brought together unintended audiences, such as automated suggestions to add existing Facebook friends on Instagram. Others found platform settings required additional steps to opt out of sharing particular kinds of information, such as the work of removing occupational information from one's Tinder profile. These technological challenges not only make it difficult to safeguard privacy, they also complicate the process of disclosing personal information and curating its degree of publicness.

At the platform level, such complications could be addressed through creative approaches that are sufficiently elastic to meet a range of user needs. Design scholar Ann Light (2011) suggests that technologies can allow for diverse and shifting discourses of identity and associated social values by queering design, applying the lens of queer theory to build in elements of fluidity, performativity, and the possibility of subversion. She proposes designs that enable user playfulness and allow for change through forgetfulness, rather than enduring data retention. Most pertinent for design-based issues of identity modulation, she argues that designers must not be afraid to "design for human diversity at the expense of machine capabilities" (p. 434), sometimes eschewing automation and algorithmic profiling for opt-in processes that give users greater control over the identities they construct and share through technology. Since these approaches make space for fluid and divergent identities, they provide room for individuals to steer their identity modulation more easily and directly.

If platforms were merely networked software applications functioning according to design principles, then it could be reasonable to expect that a few tweaks to their architecture would solve everything. However, the extent to which our personal disclosures become potentially profitable data reminds us that platforms' rigid, interconnected, template-based interfaces sustain large-scale commercial interests (Gehl, 2014; van Dijck & Poell, 2013). Previous chapters identified how design features work in tandem with platforms' markets, corporate visions, and supporting governance structures to create defaults for identity modulation. Tinder's automated importing of data to create profiles alongside norms encouraging adherence to real names enhanced personal identifiability. Instagram and

Vine amplified users' reach though content-enhancing filters and looping video within platform cultures geared toward succeeding in the attention economy. Additionally, Vine's affective intensity and relaxed policies allowed for heightened salience in identity expression.

These conditions affect users not only in their relationship to the platform but also with regard to their interpersonal, economic, and social relationships. As such, these arrangements sometimes pose complex hurdles for individuals in their identity modulation—hurdles that require attention to design as well as broader structures that impact social media users. Looking closer at each of these allows for an understanding of the multilevel changes required to impart to users greater agency over their identity modulation.

Narrow Digital Imaginaries

Chapter 2 introduced the notion of Tinder's lesbian digital imaginary, which Lindsay Ferris and I developed from our research on queer women's uses of Tinder. The lesbian digital imaginary emerged from the fusion, and consistent repetition, of queer women's cultural and digital signaling practices that were intended to be recognizable to an imagined community of similar others. To this end, queer women employed similar photographic conventions, discussion topics, and the "two women holding hands" emoji in ways that frequently referenced lesbian culture as a shorthand for identifying nonheterosexual others. While useful for deflecting the numerous heterosexual men, women, and couples who populate the app, this lesbian digital imaginary held the potential to exclude those who failed to make recognizable references to lesbian culture, those who lacked digital skills to recreate such signals, and those whose identities were not recognizable within the category of "lesbian" constructed among users. Mention of Lesbian TikTok as a boundary drawn around users alludes to a digital imaginary arising on this newer platform. Within TikTok's lesbian digital imaginary, those who have never heard of girl in red or who are unaware of platform-specific lesbian hashtags (e.g., #cottagecorelesbian) may have trouble finding and identifying as queer women on the platform, and this could be reinforced by its algorithmic silos.

It is possible for digital imaginaries to arise among other subsets of users on different platforms. Media scholar Akane Kanai's (2016) analysis of the Tumblr blog WhatShouldWeCallMe points toward a digital imaginary of readers and contributors who fused their cultural literacy of middle-class, white femininity with digital meme-making techniques to appeal to an imagined community of women united in girlfriendship. This digital imaginary could become unwelcoming toward users outside of the channeled class, race, and gender constructions as well as those who lack digital literacy concerning memes and memetic cultures of humor. Digital imaginaries are prevalent among subsets of users as boundaries constructed through shared cultural and digital aptitude that are used to demarcate those who conceive of themselves as possessing a shared identity.

Platforms can be differentially complicit in constructing a digital imaginary's boundaries. Tinder's original binary gender identifications, and the endurance of its binary profile-browsing specifications following the addition of multiple gender identities, leave little space for trans-gender users or those along a gender spectrum. This reinforces imagined perceptions of nonheterosexual female users as cisgender lesbians. Apple's inclusion of a single possible representation of a queer female relationship (if two women holding hands is not merely overlooked as being *gal pals*) contributes to its widespread circulation as an image that perpetuates normative femininity and, until recently, the erasure of those with skin tones not represented by the default yellow/white. It is likely that queer women migrating their partner seeking to platforms like TikTok that are not mainly for dating are doing so, at least in part, to avoid such baked-in gender and identity categories (Bivens & Haimson, 2016). Platforms that are moving away from automatically populating profiles with bootstrapped information—including Tinder now permitting users to log in without Facebook—hold promise for allowing users greater flexibility to write, photograph, and record themselves into being.[3]

The uneven playing field of digital literacy is often obscured by assumptions that technology use comes naturally to anyone considered to be a millennial or younger, which now comprises a large majority of social media users. However, researchers assert that the divide between people who reap personal benefits from digital technology and those who do not arises not only from access barriers but also from hindrances in learning how to skillfully use technologies (Hargittai & Hsieh, 2013). And skills deficiency can affect individuals of all ages (Eynon & Geniets, 2016). In recent years, some barriers to technology access have lessened through widespread availability and uptake of smartphones, which allow individuals to get online without investment in a home computer or WiFi. Media scholar S. Craig Watkins's (2018) ethnographic work reveals that Black, Latino, and lower-income American teens use mobile platforms for a great deal of their digital participation. However, mobile phones are often banned from the classroom in favor of one-size-fits-all educational technologies and lessons that focus on the use of basic software tools under the mandate of occupational skills development.

This approach gives little institutional support for developing digital literacy that recognizes how digital culture is co-constructed and lived. Sociologist Harry T. Dyer (2020) argues, "Technology cannot be removed from the political and social contexts in which it is so deeply embedded. Educational responses to technology similarly should not spend time and effort desperately propping up an unsustainable divide between the technological and the social" (p. 169). By keeping students' social technologies out of the classroom, schools ignore the chance to educate youth about the role of digital media in their representations of identity; social connections; and the use of digital means for enhancing their participation in broader social, economic, and political contexts. Social practices and knowledge pertaining to platforms' cultures of use must be seen as integral to digital literacy, enabling individuals to produce the kinds of media that allow them to be present in digital imaginaries. Such participation, when paired with skills for connecting interpersonally and circumventing platforms' individualizing structures, can give rise to publics and counterpublics, concretizing imagined collectives through dialogue and relationships.

A final consideration for broadening digital imaginaries' boundaries of inclusion is the need for a greater diversity of recognizable references to often marginalized identities. Many of the queer women I interviewed mentioned similar television shows, musicians, celebrities, and fashion tropes as well-known signifiers of LGBTQ culture in the Global North. Among these, *Orange Is the New Black* stood out as including representations of transgender and racialized characters. Otherwise, white, cisgender YouTubers and celebrities were most often mentioned. Normative representations of identity were recreated across social media, such as in the highly replicated lesbian digital dreamgirl images I observed on Instagram. A lacuna of queer representation was most pronounced in the music incorporated into queer women's Vines. With female rappers less prominent than male rappers on popular music charts (Mohammed-baksh & Callison, 2015) and a scarcity of popular, queer female artists, queer women often chose to lip-sync to songs by male rappers. Where queer representation exists in media, participants were more likely to draw on cisgender, white, and often feminine representations of lesbian identity that remain prominent across television, film, and streaming media. When queer representation was missing altogether, they had to get creative.

However, the landscape of media representation is continually changing. We may be witnessing an effective shift toward more LGBTQ representations of racialized and gender-diverse people, such as through the mainstream popularity of television shows like *Pose* (2018–2021) and queer musicians like Princess Nokia. This shift has the potential to generate an increased number of signifiers that transgender, gender nonconforming, and racialized queer women can draw on in their representations of identity as references that are now more widely recognizable. Beyond this, the greater the reach and salience of a diversity of queer female social media users, the more others are likely to encounter representations that decenter normative identities. In this mutually reinforcing process, user agency in identity modulation can fuel the circulation of identity representations that enable others' identity modulation.

Burnout before Microcelebrity Status

Chapter 3's exploration of identity modulation in service of self-branding revealed multiple modes of labor involved in constructing a marketable persona. The intensity and conditions of this work contributed to some queer women's feelings of exploitation and alienation as they shared personal content to form relationships with their audiences. Although some women experienced benefits in the form of greater social capital—which may eventually translate into economic capital through an increase in clients, buyers, or eventual brand partnerships—compensation for their labor remained indirect and obscure. These women's experiences are congruent with the explosion of influencer-generated media and news coverage pertaining to burnout in the influencer industry. Several influencers blame their burnout on labor conditions that include the need to constantly produce, relate to one's audience, navigate the threat of algorithmic invisibility, and deal with harassment from viewers (Parkin, 2018). Many of the women I spoke with also faced these problems, even without thousands of followers.

Despite past optimism that social media would lower barriers to entry for everyday creative production (Jenkins et al., 2013), the economic conditions of platformed production tend to reinforce and intensify inequalities. Media scholar Kylie Jarrett (2015) identifies the role of gender in how digital labor is often undervalued and left uncompensated. She notes that much of the affective, relational, and information-based work conducted through digital technologies is immaterial, in that it does not directly involve the production of material goods. Immaterial labor—especially domestic labor that is often thought of as "women's work"—is often unpaid or poorly compensated. She explains, "Thus, not only do the immaterial aspects of domestic labour bear resemblance to the kinds of value-producing contributions associated with digital media consumers, unpaid domestic work also articulates the tension between agency and exploitation that animates the politics of digital media" (p. 11). Queer women discussed in this book exercised agency in self-branding and building potentially lucrative connections on Instagram and Vine, doing so without the surveillance of a manager or restrictions imposed by a company. However, some also experienced exploitation in the form of undervalued, unrecognized labor that seemed to have little payoff. Jarrett's association of invisible, unpaid domestic labor with digital cultural production relates to scholars' observations that women's microcelebrity labor is not seen as supporting an actual career and yet is expected to be given freely (or provided in exchange for freebies) (Abidin, 2016; Duffy, 2017). More generally, women's digital self-representation is often disregarded as unimportant and narcissistic (Senft & Baym, 2015). Across sectors, jobs that are seen as constituting the kind of reproductive (e.g., cleaning, child care) and affective (e.g., service, administration) labor that our society has long associated with womanhood are less compensated than others that are understood to be within a masculine realm of material production. Therefore, the devaluation of women's immaterial labor spreads out to the influencer industry overall, being work comprised of affective relationship maintenance and the reproduction of digital content, broadly hindering anyone's ability to make a stable living through social media.

Within this context of gendered labor inequalities, platforms and commercial intermediaries bring new complications to the relationships that must be negotiated through this labor. Platforms have enormous power to shift the rules for success when they rapidly change financial and algorithmic incentive structures. For example, YouTube's "tiered governance strategy" (Caplan & Gillespie, 2020) allows certain users, such as prominent media personalities, to function under more lenient restrictions than amateur creators. Just as YouTubers attempt to circumnavigate these rules governing algorithmic visibility and monetization, many queer women whom I interviewed tried to maintain or extend their reach despite platform reconfigurations that threatened the circulation of their content. Their approaches included shout-outs to popular users and defiant posting of attention-garnering content, such as Queenie's seminude burlesque photos, which were rewarded by audiences if not by platform policies.

Within this ever-shifting platform landscape, creators attempting to monetize their social media often aim for brand partnerships and sponsored posts—labor for which there is no standardized compensation. In response to uneven pay, especially for LGBTQ and racialized creators, influencers have turned to Instagram accounts like @InfluencerPayGap to anonymously share pay rates (Ashley, 2020). More formal efforts are taking shape to pressure brand intermediaries to pay fair wages, such as the creation of unions and trade associations like the American Influencer Council. Through these responses, aspiring and established influencers challenge the uneven and discriminatory labor relations that currently give a disproportionate amount of power to platforms and brands.

The formation of unions and coalitions of people whose social media production constitutes labor has a strong potential for changing platformed conditions of work. These entities counteract exactly what makes this kind of labor so alienating: individualized entrepreneurialism. Platform infrastructures support the formation of individualized networks, in which the individual features as the central node in their friend or follower relationships (Rainie & Wellman, 2012). This positions individuals as solely responsible for maintaining relationships with their audiences, giving rise to solitary influencers who make it big—not groups or communities. As such, influencers assume the role of the enterprising entrepreneur, left to manage every facet of their careers (Duffy & Wissinger, 2017). This individualism fuels the kind of competitiveness that made Chrissy tired of Viners creating content only to be discovered for brand sponsorships and not in service of fostering community or public dialogue. Entrepreneurialism also makes individuals responsible for their risk of failure, heightening the stakes of labor channeled into social media production. It is no wonder that Jaxx felt like she was putting herself on the line when pressured to produce appealing content. She was responding to the platform and labor structures that make individuals responsible for their social and economic success without any guarantees or safety nets.

Patchwork Platform Governance

In chapter 4, I connected the censorship and harassment queer women experienced on Instagram and Vine to platform governance approaches that are uneven and inconsistent in their application. Thinking this through with Jean Burgess and Nicolas Suzor, we understood this as patchwork platform governance that upholds seemingly robust policies and procedures of content moderation without attending to how platform features and cultures of use impact who is actually protected. Such governance approaches often rely on the co-moderation of content, with users playing an active role in flagging posts that may or may not be reviewed by platform employees before consequences are applied. This governance takes a *patchwork* form because it seeks to enforce evolving rules of content removal and user policing without addressing toxic technocultures that harness the same policies and technical structures to target vulnerable user groups.

What is the gaping hole in such governance approaches? It is the failure of companies like Facebook and Reddit to acknowledge and take responsibility for how platforms contribute to cultures of use, including those that harass, discriminate, and threaten other users. By ignoring such cultures, platforms act as though they are neutral conduits while arbitrating which content and communities flourish online (Gillespie, 2015). Countering freedom-of-speech arguments that attempt to justify platforms' minimal action on user harassment, Suzor (2019) argues in favor of stepping in: "Because doing nothing means tolerating hateful speech that will inevitably silence and further marginalize already-marginalized voices, doing nothing is not a neutral policy" (p. 136). Doing nothing is, in fact, a policy that paves the way for a great deal of harm toward vulnerable users and can drive them from a platform.

Several scholars have suggested how platforms could refine their governance approaches to better protect marginalized users. Their recommendations range from increasing the transparency of moderation processes (Suzor, 2019), to paying moderators a decent wage with benefits instead of outsourcing moderation as underpaid, precarious clickwork (Roberts, 2019), to curtailing forms of algorithmic governance that can amplify biased, racist, and sexist content (Gerrard & Thornham, 2020; Matamoros-Fernández, 2017). Certainly, such changes would make a difference in the experiences of the women I interviewed. Transparent moderation processes would offer individuals like Alex greater recourse when policy-abiding photos are flagged for seemingly no reason other than homophobia. No matter who conducts moderation, it needs to be carried out with specificity that recognizes existing inequalities and how they become transferred to platform environments. Clickworkers with little knowledge of localized sociopolitical contexts are unlikely to be able to apply such fine-tuned judgment, nor are they paid enough to do so. As seen in the case of Instagram's censorship of #lesbian, algorithmic moderation is often too broad and blunt an instrument to capture this specificity, wiping out swathes of intimate and meaningful content while still being gamed by pornographic spammers. Tumblr's algorithmic enforcement of its ban on nudity also provides evidence of this, as users' photos including clothed selfies, drawings of reptiles, and even a vase have been flagged as explicit (Krishna, 2018). Informed, human-led governance processes to which users are privy would improve upon the current patchwork. Scholars have begun to mull over possibilities for greater, more democratic involvement on the part of users and civil society as key actors in these governance processes (Gillespie, 2018; Suzor, 2019).

Most powerfully, scholars and the public alike are calling on social media companies to cast aside pretenses of neutrality when it comes to hate and harmful activity conducted through their platforms. Many popular platforms are headquartered in the United States and protected under Section 230 of the Communications Decency Act, which provides them with "safe harbor" as entities not legally responsible for the content users post, giving them the choice of whether and how much to moderate content (Gillespie, 2018). However, Tarleton Gillespie (2018) observes that as platforms have become highly influential in public discourse, they now "inhabit a position of responsibility—not only to individual users but to the public they powerfully affect" (p. 208). Gillespie calls on platforms to move from cleaning up messes in an ad hoc manner to instead begin assuming the role of custodians who recognize their social responsibility to uphold civic values, and he invites users to hold platforms to this standard.

Dangerous developments have slowly led some platforms to take greater responsibility for user actions and content. For example, after a violent clash between white nationalists and protestors in Charlottesville, Virginia, Facebook and Reddit banned several far-right and neo-Nazi communities (Little & Hollister, 2017), recognizing that their platforms gave these communities a place to connect, flourish, and strategize. Subsequently, Reddit has introduced new policies leading to the banning of several subreddits, including r/The_Donald, a community of Donald Trump supporters also known for posting violent and hateful content that frequently violates the platform's policies while also antagonizing other user communities (Newton, 2020). The new policy goes beyond previous steps of "quarantining" r/The_Donald by preventing its content from being featured on Reddit's homepage and requiring users to read a warning before joining the subreddit. Leaving behind these weaker measures, Reddit has finally dropped its neutral stance through new rules explicitly stating that "communities and users that promote hate based on identity or vulnerability will be banned." Additionally, Reddit specifies, "Debate and creativity are welcome, but spam and malicious attempts to interfere with other communities are not" (Spez, 2020). These rules very clearly prohibit hate speech and targeted harassment, providing Reddit with the impetus to purge several communities guilty of this behavior from its platform.

There are indications that Reddit's new policy is part of a larger reckoning for platforms concerning their responsibility to protect users from harmful misinformation and foster public discourse that does not incite hate, discrimination, or violence. Donald Trump's social media activity, particularly that which he carried out while President of the United States, challenged platforms to act in the best interests of vulnerable populations and democracy more broadly. Following several instances in which Twitter and Facebook made judgment calls about moderating presidential posts, such as those spreading misinformation (Mangan & Breuninger, 2020) and threatening Black Lives Matter protestors (Feiner, 2020), these platforms eventually banned Trump's accounts altogether. Deeming his posts to have contributed to the violent protests at the US Capitol on January 6, 2021, they removed Trump as a preventative measure against future violent uprisings. While Twitter's ban was permanent (Twitter Inc., 2021), Facebook deferred the issue to its Oversight Board, a Facebook-appointed—yet purportedly independent—decision-making body that proposes nonbinding recommendations to Facebook through an appeals process. In June 2021, Facebook adopted the Oversight Board's recommendation to ban Trump for two years and to further assess "whether the risk to public safety has receded" (Clegg, 2021) before reinstating his account in the future. This action against a former president could be seen as addressing some element of patchwork governance: it removes the voice of someone who was arguably a leader and icon to right-wing, nationalist toxic technocultures.

However, this decision was ad hoc, with Facebook admitting that it "did not have enforcement protocols in place adequate to respond to such unusual events" (Clegg, 2021). Despite this claim, only Trump's status as a US president was unusual in this instance, as leaders and governments of other countries have often been complicit in using the platform to share misinformation and hate speech in support of violence (Bengali, 2021). Facebook's lack of action prior to widespread public scrutiny (specifically, concerning US politics) reflects how its governance remains patchy, as it is only triggered within certain conditions. Further, while these platforms have specific protocols pertaining to content produced by politicians and world leaders, there is little to systematically protect others from the toxic technocultures they stir up and that endure even in their absence. Banning those who incite violence and hate is only a partial solution, while steps must be taken to support the marginalized communities targeted by such hate. Quite the opposite happens when their posts are still regularly removed and censored, as reflected in earlier chapters and countless other instances.[4]

Identity modulation has positive outcomes for individuals in their relationships, self-branding, and public participation when people are able to express diverse identities in ways that are not exploited or met with discrimination and harassment. By unpacking each of these complex challenges for individuals in steering their identity modulation, it is possible to see that changes need to take place on multiple levels. These include platform-level interventions that attend to infrastructure, markets, and governance (Nieborg & Poell, 2018), noting not only how algorithms and digital interfaces shape individuals' self-representations but also how users are greatly impacted by platforms' financial interests and governance approaches. They also involve scrutiny of our evolving labor relations, as precarious, individualized gig work becomes an increasingly common mode of working, enabled through digital technologies. Additionally, there is a need to look at broader cultural representations that shape public discourse, identifying where greater diversity is required so that a wider range of identities becomes recognizable while ensuring that hate speech and discrimination do not punish people for making such identities salient.

These big-picture changes at the levels of technology, economy, and culture are important—they require attention and, with so many moving parts, are prone to slow change. This book and its findings support the many scholars pressing against specific issues of platform infrastructure, markets, and governance to uncover further insights into why and how such changes must be realized. In wrapping up, I want to provide a reframing of identity modulation that could galvanize change—at multiple levels and speeds—as it makes apparent how we are all affected by constraints on our digital self-representation.

IDENTITY MODULATION AS A RIGHT WITHIN DIGITAL CITIZENSHIP

Arrangements identified in the previous section hindered identity modulation because they constrained individuals' agency in adjusting the personal identifiability, reach, and salience of their digital self-representations. Agency is lost when narrow digital imaginaries constrain the range of salient identities people can express. Exploitative labor conditions hamper individuals' reach and require them to work harder to circulate their self-brands. Patchwork platform governance imperils users when their personally identifiable information puts them at risk of targeted harassment and doxxing by members of toxic technocultures who go unchecked by platforms' moderation mechanisms. Identity modulation is a process that users and platforms negotiate together, but such arrangements curtail individuals' influence in this process. On top of these broader hindrances to identity modulation, queer women spoke specifically of the difficulties they encountered in representing sexual identity, including struggles to craft desired representations and express them to particular audiences and not others.

It is not surprising that sexual identity, in particular, is difficult for individuals to modulate in platform contexts. There has been a broad deplatforming of sexual content over the past several years, as social media companies aim to appease laws like FOSTA-SESTA[5] that implicate platforms as liable for sex trafficking (Tiidenberg & van der Nagel, 2020). Resulting from the overly broad reach of anti-sex-trafficking laws, which are often applied to consensual sex work and other sexual activities, platforms have ramped up their regulation of sexual content and related communities (Liu, 2021). Social media scholars Katrin Tiidenberg and Emily van der Nagel (2020) identify three key mechanisms through which this deplatforming is carried out: platform moderation that enforces rules banning sexual content, affordances that constrain user choices concerning sexual expression, and algorithms that determine the visibility of sexual content. These mechanisms are resonant in queer women's experiences of censorship through moderation, limited affordances for sexual self-representation, and algorithmic influence on the reach of their content related to sexuality and sexual identity. Such platform mechanisms are not only congruent with US laws, they reflect what media studies scholars Susanna Paasonen, Kylie Jarrett, and Ben Light (2019) identify as a combination of corporate conservatism and residual Puritan *structures of feeling*, building on the work of Raymond Williams (1977). They argue that an American Puritan cultural legacy remains ingrained in societal associations and norms relating to sex, contributing to platforms' "seemingly automatic association of unsafety with sex" (p. 169). Through their study of content hashtagged #NSFW (not safe for work), they observe how "safety" has broadly "become a euphemism for the policy of filtering out or limiting access to sexual content online" (p. 9). This leads to hypervigilance in the policing of sexual content as our platforms are progressively scrubbed clean, leaving fewer sexual outlets online.

A defense of sexual content and rebuke of platform censorship may come across as contradictory, given my previous assertion that platforms should indeed act to protect their users. However, Paasonen et al. (2019) argue, "As constitutive elements of ways of being in the world, sex and sexuality are not inherently either safe or unsafe" (p. 171). Sex can indeed be used to harm, especially when it is forced upon individuals, as in the unsolicited dick pics many of my interviewees encountered in DMs (direct messages). Rather, consent is key to the vibrant sexual cultures that many individuals enjoy online (Paasonen et al., 2019). As we have seen in these pages, agentically created and consensually viewed self-representations of sexuality and sexual identity—from sexy selfies to thirst traps—contribute to individuals' sense of self, connections with others, and participation in publics. This content clearly warrants different treatment from hate speech and threats of violence. However, platform policies often lump everything together in their moderation.

Early in 2020, I was fortunate to attend a talk in which Susanna Paasonen discussed where we could go from here.[6] She pointed to the possibility that platform governance could be guided by the recognition of individuals' sexual rights, as a subset of their human rights. This makes a lot of sense, as it connects to long-standing and newer developments in thinking about sexual citizenship. Sociologist Diane Richardson (1998) highlights that sexual citizenship is a term with multiple and shifting definitions, since citizenship can be understood through multiplicities, such as civil, political, and social rights; belonging to a nation; and consumer participation. She considers how such elements of citizenship have often been most accessible to heterosexuals and men. Indeed, much feminist and LGBTQ organizing in the late twentieth and twenty-first centuries has focused on establishing women and nonheterosexuals as citizens with full participation in politics and society as well as consumer and civil life. In her more recent book, Richardson (2018) dedicates a section to discussing sexual rights in relation to sexual citizenship. She establishes three main framings for sexual rights: "conduct-based" (e.g., to participate in sexual activity, enjoy pleasure, have bodily self-determination); "identity-based" (e.g., self-expression and self-definition); and "relationship-based" (e.g., choice of sexual partners, public recognition and civil rights granted to relationships). It is possible to understand the queer women in this book as engaging in identity modulation to exercise their sexual rights. Their intimate disclosures comprised of flirting on Tinder could be seen as precursors to sexual conduct. Their self-definition across platforms exercised identity-based rights while showcasing relationships on Instagram and Vine was one element that garnered public recognition and reflected participation more broadly in social, economic, and public facets of life.

But platforms can pose obstacles to enacting these rights and accessing sexual citizenship. Scholars observe how digital technologies greatly shape our participation in politics, markets, and society, characterizing a form of digital citizenship (Mossberger et al., 2008). This notion of digital citizenship is much debated, as it has been steeped in optimism that digital technologies will open up new routes of participation and give voice to those previously unheard (Couldry, 2010). In actuality, digital citizenship is a site of control by institutions and platforms, of contest as users challenge these governing bodies, and of emergent cultures as individuals and communities define participation on their own terms (Vivienne et al., 2016). Media scholar Kath Albury (2016) brings sexual and digital citizenship into dialogue when she asks, "If the notion of digital citizenship implies recognition of one's rights and responsibilities in online and mobile-mediated spaces, how does the notion of sexual citizenship intersect with and extend these rights and responsibilities?" (p. 214). She discusses "digital sexual citizenship" (p. 226) as a negotiation among users, technologies, and institutions that recognizes freedom from sexual- and gender-related abuse but also, importantly, people's entitlement to sexual self-representation. Scholars argue that the sexual rights inherent to such citizenship can be protected through "contextual moderation approaches and the centrality of user consent" (Spišak et al., 2021, p. 2). Platforms must gauge the context for sexual expressions, which individuals work so hard to tailor through identity modulation. Mutual collaboration between platforms and users in building contextual boundaries allows for appropriate audiences to receive sexual content. Additional technological mechanisms can provide individual users within these audiences with the final say in whether to view it or not. Therefore, preserving digital sexual citizenship requires platforms to bolster user agency in identity modulation while becoming as sensitive to context as many of their users already are.

These intersections between sexual citizenship and digital citizenship provide fuel for the argument that identity modulation is too important to leave in the hands of platforms and their default arrangements. Although this book has focused on identity modulation in the disclosure of sexual identity, similar processes of adjusting personal identifiability, reach, and salience are pivotal to the management of a range of personal information. This management is especially pertinent when disclosing that which is often subject to stigma in our society, such as employment status, physical or mental ability, education level, income, and many other qualities that we share differently across contexts. These personal elements can be thought of as comprising the intimate, broadly described by sociologist Ken Plummer (2003) as a "complex sphere of 'inmost' relationships with the self and others" (p. 13). Plummer adds another layer to the myriad definitions of citizenship, identifying intimate citizenship as "the decisions people have to make over *the control (or not) over* one's body, feelings, relationships; *access (or not) to* representations, relationships, public spaces, etc.; and *socially grounded choices (or not) about* identities, gender experiences, erotic experiences" (p. 14; emphasis in original). These facets of intimate citizenship easily encompass sexuality but also include other elements of the self and one's relationships, which are often viewed as private. Plummer understands intimate citizenship as a bridge between the personal and the political, through which the intimate is brought into and shapes publics.

Updating this concept for a digital context, media scholar Son Vivienne (2016b) introduces intimate citizenship 3.0 as "constitutive digitally mediated practices that intersect across intimacy, privacy, publicness and difference" (p. 147). This concept emerges from Vivienne's work with gender-diverse communities, noting their strategies for participating in intimate citizenship through networked publics, with "3.0" highlighting the seamlessness of their offline and online lives. Several strategies of intimate citizenship 3.0 that Vivienne observes, such as using "a platform for speaking across difference" and the "curation of privacy through selective self-representation" (p. 157), resemble actions that the queer women discussed in this book took through identity modulation. More specifically, identity modulation involves the curation of publicness in order to participate in intimate citizenship. These strategies are conducted by what Vivienne calls "everyday activists," meaning ordinary people whose everyday expressions of identity challenge perceived social norms. Pivotally, the enactment of everyday activism through intimate citizenship 3.0 "constitutes an intervention—a strategic and targeted experiment in catalyzing erosive change" (Vivienne, 2016a, p. 210). The digital circulation of intimate expressions, historically and often still relegated to the private sphere, to a broad range of audiences has a slow but noticeable effect on changing ways of thinking. Identity modulation is crucial to this circulation, as it constitutes the way intimate disclosures are represented and managed.

Since identity modulation is integral to intimate citizenship 3.0, which can be understood as a subset of digital citizenship more broadly, it follows that individual agency over identity modulation should be included in calls for platforms and associated institutions to preserve and respect human rights as digital rights. Suzor (2019) makes a compelling argument that platforms should draw on standards provided by international human rights law, embedding its principles into their operations. He underscores: "The core rights—guarantees of freedom of expression, privacy, equality, and so on—are values that express a common international agreement about the protections all people are entitled to" (p. 131). As this book has made clear, identity modulation does not quite fit under the category of privacy, as it deals with adjustments to publicness. Nor is it merely about expression, as it has to do with managing how these expressions are received and by whom. It is instead about modulating one's personal identifiability, reach, and salience in instances of intimate disclosure so as to reinstate context. In the sense that identity modulation is necessary for digital participation in relationships, publics, and counterpublics, it must be counted as a human right protected under one's digital citizenship.

DOING SOMETHING DIFFERENT

In the midst of Canada's initial COVID-19 pandemic lockdown measures, I reached for artist Jenny Odell's (2019) book, *How to Do Nothing: Resisting the Attention Economy.* I was surprised to find that her book, instead of reinforcing the inclination to hide under my desk until the crisis subsided, was actually a call to action—a call for a different kind of action. Odell expresses frustration with the paucity of connection she observes as being possible on social media due to context collapse. Although I have described many queer women's meaningful connections rendered through platforms, Odell's laments about the loss of our ability to be fully present with others in time and space resonate with the effort these women put into identity modulation to overcome these hindrances. She suggests that one way forward is to embrace the opposite of the ever-expanding ideology of manifest destiny undergirding current economic and political aims, taking an approach of "manifest dismantling" as an intentional undoing of the systems and structures that bind us (p. 190). That we return to nothingness when current arrangements no longer serve people in their everyday lives.

Having explored several avenues for change in this last chapter, I can see how manifest dismantling may be one way to respond to the state of social media. In combination with Ann Light's (2011) assertion that people should be valued over machine capabilities, it seems apparent that some networked connections inherent to platforms must necessarily be dismantled. Connections between and within platforms that stymie individuals' ability to modulate their reach, and connections that convey personal identifiability when it is unwanted, need to be made optional or removed altogether. Manifest dismantling of platform arrangements could also look like discarding policies that treat sex and nudity as unsafe, starting from scratch with consent and sexual citizenship as central principles. Platform incentivization programs and brands that expect individuals to give their labor for free, especially those underpaying LGBTQ and racialized creators, warrant dismantling, as they fail to value people's personal and creative production in equitable ways.

However, Odell does not merely stop at dismantling. She also calls for attention and rebuilding. When it comes to social media, she too arrives at the need to address context collapse through a form of "context collection" as the "restoration of context" via arrangements that enable people to speak effectively to "the right people (or person) at the right time" (p. 176). I have highlighted how providing individuals with greater agency to modulate their personal identifiability, reach, and salience of personal disclosure allows for this restoration of context. Indeed, it enables individuals to carve out a particular digital context for their self-representations, drawing on the opportunities provided by platforms' digital affordances. However, platform arrangements of technology, markets, and governance shape whether individuals can reinstate context through identity modulation. Since platforms are embedded within broader economic, political, and cultural landscapes, contributions toward wider change are needed in order to make a difference at the personal level of individual agency. Odell also recognizes that manifest dismantling works hand in hand with people attending to not only technological design but also other areas of importance, such as labor rights, women's rights, and antiracist initiatives. She reassures us: "As in any ecology, the fruits of our efforts within any of these fields may well reach beyond to the others" (p. 199).

As such, I see the findings shared throughout *Personal but Not Private* as pointing toward the possibility of both fast and slow change. Some adjustments to provide individuals with greater agency over identity modulation could take effect quite quickly, especially at the design level. For example, platforms could easily broaden their features and categories for self-representation. They could alter moderation algorithms that overcensor queer content and women's bodies as swiftly as other updates that prioritize the visibility of some media producers over others. However, such fixes would only be motivated by, and become fully effective through, broader systemic changes to the larger issues this chapter has outlined.

Even so, change at any level provides a chance to break out of repetition—the repetition of stereotypes, exploitation, and platforms preserving their interests while neglecting their responsibility to users and the public more generally. This repetition is evident in the similar networked arrangements that abound across platforms and even in newer ones. As I highlighted in the chapter's introduction, TikTok seems to be replicating the application of selective governance policies and algorithmic structures that have served the interests of other popular platforms but not necessarily their users. Initial changes that grant greater agency to people over their identity modulation can lead to longer-term, higher-level changes as individuals' digital self-representation has the capacity to impact social, cultural, political, and economic constraints on digital citizenship. As Vivienne (2016a) underscores, intimate citizenship 3.0 contributes to erosive change by bringing personal lives into public view, challenging the status quo. By steering identity modulation processes in order to participate fully as digital citizens, a wide diversity of people can contribute to and convene around public discourse. And public discourse, after all, is "poetic world making" (Warner, 2002, p. 114) as it seeks to characterize and realize new worlds. This book has shown how queer women's public discourse, in the form of digital self-representation and disclosures of sexual identity, gives rise to publics and counterpublics with the potential to realize change and invoke new ways of being.

I still remember that as I interviewed Chrissy about her Vines, it was daytime in Australia, but across the ocean the sun was setting through her living room window. As her ten-year-old daughter wandered over and waved at me through the webcam, our conversation turned to discussion of why Chrissy was out and active on social media. Her words encapsulated the process of world making: "Some people can't live with themselves because the whole world is condemning us for being who we are. So, you've got to fight back somehow. And there's people like me that are comfortable being—I'm comfortable being me. So, it helps them put themselves at ease and say, 'I can be myself without feeling like the world is against me.'" Through identity modulation, her digital self-representation as a Black, lesbian wife and mother characterizes a world where people experiencing discrimination and marginalization can instead feel at ease.

Platforms have a choice of whether or not they will be hospitable to these worlds. And they have a range of scholarship to draw from in terms of how they can become responsible hosts to a diversity of people, communities, and publics. However, it is certain that if identity modulation becomes untenable on a platform, queer women will continue to find new outlets for convening publics and enacting their world making. Whether on TikTok or somewhere else, they will mobilize the digital tools and cultural signals available to establish relationships, access social and economic capital, and make powerful statements about their right to participate in society. Since people can realize such outcomes through identity modulation, which makes possible intimate and impactful personal disclosures, changes to platforms and their broader ecologies should restore to individuals the volume control for their digital self-representation.

Methods of the Study

As discussed in chapter 1, this research took place from 2014 to 2017 through a mixed-methods approach that combined digital research methods with more traditional social science methods. For Tinder, Instagram, and Vine, I analyzed user content, individuals' experiences, and the platform's role in shaping these. To investigate that role, I applied the walkthrough method to each platform as "a way of engaging directly with an app's interface to examine its technological mechanisms and embedded cultural references to understand how it guides users and shapes their experiences" (Light et al., 2018, p. 882). The walkthrough method consists of two components: establishing the environment of expected use and performing the technical walkthrough. An app's environment of expected use is comprised of its vision, operating model, and governance policies. For each platform in this study, I established its environment of expected use by collecting and analyzing official company materials (e.g., web pages, blog posts, and social media accounts) as well as articles from trade press and media coverage. The technical walkthrough involves stepping through registration, everyday use, and discontinuation or leaving an app, paying close attention to its interface arrangement, functions and features, textual content and tone, and symbolic representation (pp. 891–892). I conducted initial technical walkthroughs of each app early in the study and then carried out subsequent walkthroughs when major software updates occurred. I used my Apple iPhone for these walkthroughs, as it was my available device at the time. Overall, the walkthrough method provided a sense of how each platform's technological, social, economic, and governance-related arrangements sought to guide users in their activity, providing the default arrangements for identity modulation that users encountered, engaged with, and resisted.

My other methods were shaped by attention to the medium specificity of each platform (Bucher & Helmond, 2017; Rogers, 2013), heeding differential opportunities for data collection as well as ethical concerns. I approached Tinder with particular caution, since it is widely perceived to be a dating and hook-up app, with users sharing intimate data pertaining to these activities (Albury et al., 2017). Tinder profiles are also only viewable through the creation of an account, presuming that users are on the platform for a similar purpose. For these reasons, I did not conduct large-scale analysis of queer women's profile content. Instead, I asked the women I interviewed to provide screenshots of their profile information and photos. Although other researchers have recruited interviewees in-app (Ward, 2016), I felt that Tinder's swipe encouraged matching without reading profile details and that I could not be sure how widely my profile would be circulated by Tinder's algorithm. Instead, I recruited interview participants through LGBTQ Facebook groups and social media networks.

Overall, I interviewed ten female Tinder users ranging from nineteen to thirty-five years old, eight located in Australia and two in Canada. Participants self-described their sexual identity, identifying as gay, lesbian, bisexual, queer, and "homoflexible" (alternating between bisexual, pansexual, or gay). Despite the variation among participants with respect to these qualities as well as occupation and level of schooling, all identified as white. This could be for many reasons, including the dominant whiteness of LGBTQ spaces and the rampant racism on dating apps, which may dissuade racialized people from using them or participating in research about them. While I should have continued recruiting participants to address this serious limitation, time and funding constraints prohibited me from doing so. Although this aspect of my sample enabled a critique of the whiteness of symbols circulated as part of Tinder's lesbian digital imaginary (see chapter 2), these findings should be read in tandem with the work of scholars who explore racialized people's experiences on dating apps, including Sarah Adeyinka-Skold, Bronwyn Carlson, and Emerich Daroya. I asked participants to choose pseudonyms, given the intimate context of Tinder and that we were discussing their dating lives, and some chose creative options as seen in the text. With interviews taking place in person or over videoconference as per participants' preferences, I asked them to guide me on a walkthrough of their accounts and Tinder use, similar to the scrollback method in which participants coanalyze their digital traces (Robards & Lincoln, 2017).

Collecting user data and approaching individuals for interviews was different on Instagram and Vine, two platforms whose users posted publicly available content depicting a range of subject matter. Available data are not, by default, public data (Franzke et al., 2019; Zimmer, 2010), but the content posted to public accounts using popular hashtags is often intended to be seen by many users. I focused on the most popular hashtags (i.e., those with the largest number of posts) related to queer female identity on each platform, analyzing user posts to identify key themes. At the time, Instagram's application programming interface (API) was compatible with the Instagram Hashtag Explorer housed by the Digital Methods Initiative at the University of Amsterdam and programmed by new media scholar Bernhard Rieder. This tool has since been rendered ineffective, as Rieder's (2016) attempts to clear the review process Instagram introduced in 2016 were unsuccessful, drawing into question how researchers can access social media data at scale for the public good. In 2015, using this tool allowed me to analyze just over four hundred posts from twenty hashtags. Although the tool also retrieved numerous pornographic images, these could be considered commercial spam, and their visual content was not examined in depth except as an influence on Instagram's visual landscape and governance policies, which I address in chapter 4. Facing a lack of such tools for Vine, I manually collected post data (e.g., date created, URL, caption, and hashtags) in a spreadsheet for seventy-seven Vines from seven popular LGBTQ hashtags, which were dominated by queer women.

The broader analysis of user content also served as a way to recruit interview participants from Instagram and Vine. I identified posts created by individuals (not organizations or businesses) and sent direct messages with an invitation to participate in the study. One strength of this approach was that it allowed me to contact individuals who were outside my networks and might not be reached by standard recruitment through LGBTQ organizations. However, even women who agreed to interviews told me I was lucky they had read my invitation, since they were accustomed to deleting messages from people they did not already know. The apps reinforced this response, filtering messages outside of their main inboxes. After sending numerous messages, six Instagrammers and two Viners agreed to interviews, with another two Instagrammers responding to a call I subsequently sent out through social media groups and networks. The lack of participation from Viners coincided with the platform's dwindling numbers by the time I was conducting interviews. After examining interviews separately, I chose to make sense of the eight Instagram and two Vine interviews together in order to compare and contrast these women's experiences, practices, and responses to similar and different platform influences.

All ten of these participants had public accounts on the platforms and welcomed me to analyze their posts. As they were spread across different countries, including Australia, Canada, Thailand, and the United States, interviews took place over telephone or videoconference, and I asked participants to speak in depth about their platform activity, combining the scrollback method (Robards & Lincoln, 2017) with photo elicitation (Harper, 2002) as we discussed their images. Participants ranged in age, from twenty-four to forty-six, and in occupation, although, as I note in chapter 3, many were self-employed or engaged in work where they needed to build a personal brand. Participants also included two individuals identifying as African American; one as Latina; one as Thai; one as mixed Hawaiian, Chinese, Filipino, and white; and one as mixed Japanese and white, with the rest identifying as white. They identified as lesbian, gay, and bisexual. With all self-identifying as women during the study, one participant identified as transfemale, one as genderqueer, and one as gender nonconforming.

A small number of participants have subsequently come out as nonbinary individuals or as transgender men in the years since the study was conducted. I have maintained the gender and pronouns they used during our interviews in order to analyze their self-representations within this particular context in their biographical history. However, I wish to clarify that doing so does not stem from an intention to erase gender diversity or to use incorrect pronouns for research participants. Instead, I recognize that digital self-representation has been integral to the survival and flourishing of transgender and nonbinary people, and I wish to point readers in the direction of growing scholarship in this area, such as work by Andre Cavalcante, Thomas J. Billard, Oliver Haimson, Tobias Raun, and Son Vivienne. Rapidly changing forms of gender representation in combination with digital platforms' affordances and constraints also warrant much future scholarly attention to the experiences of transgender and nonbinary people.

I provided the choice of using a pseudonym or their username, and several participants chose to go by their username, likely due to the public nature of their accounts and because accruing followers is a central aim of participation on Instagram and Vine. However, given that this book's publication comes several years following these interviews, I have opted to use truncated or modified versions of these usernames. I have taken this step in an attempt to prevent the potential context collapse of participants' past self-representations becoming conflated with their present-day self-representations through search engine algorithms or other automated mechanisms that may connect their mention here with their accounts. While their accounts could still be identified with effort, I am mindful of the propensity of a published book to bring more attention to their past self-representations than they may have considered at the time of providing consent. I believe this measure to be part of a feminist ethics of care approach, which digital media scholars Mary Elizabeth Luka and Mélanie Millette (2018) note is key to recognizing that social media data are shaped by power relationships. They underscore "paying attention to how our research may affect those under study" (p. 4) to ask how researchers can responsibly disseminate their findings. Given that this book emphasizes giving people the space for fluidity of identity and agency over how they show up to different audiences, these modified usernames are an effort to support this within the evolving digital landscape and across personal changes that participants have undergone over time.

I made sense of the mixed materials from platforms, users, and interviews through multiple forms of analysis. I conducted textual (McKee, 2003) and visual (Rose, 2012) analysis of user content, coding and recoding images to identify emergent themes. I also performed multiple rounds of coding of interview transcripts, iteratively applying descriptive, topical, and analytic codes and developing thematic code trees (Morse & Richards, 2002; Richards, 2009). Most of my analysis of platform walkthrough materials came together through writing (Pelias, 2011) and rewriting about how elements of the environment of expected use were concretized in platform infrastructures. I further synthesized the higher-level themes from each approach in a multitude of collegial discussions, conference presentations, and writings that have been pivotal precursors to this book.

I have had ample time to locate and reflect upon my role in relation to this research. It is quite clear that the study's motivations stem from my personal experiences of digitally mediated self-representation and that this shaped my research decisions, such as the apps examined, and my ability to reach out to participants through these apps and LGBTQ networks. Some shared positionality with research participants can simultaneously afford insider status and allow for deeper understanding of their accounts while also making it tempting to project upon them or make assumptions about their experiences (Berger, 2015). Indeed, it helped that I had seen *Orange Is the New Black*, knew about Kristen Stewart's coming out process, and followed Ruby Rose fan accounts across Instagram and Vine—not to mention that my agility with the study's apps made the walkthroughs easier than if they had been completely unfamiliar. However, I had to work to see these apps as "strange" again to notice functionalities I initially overlooked and how others' use was different from mine. I also listened closely to participants for what was unique about their experiences on these apps and to fully understand their rich journeys relating to sexual identity and coming out over years and decades. I kept their accounts in perspective through my broader analysis of queer women's social media posts. I too have been on a journey; I am no longer panicked posting about my sexual identity the way I was in 2012, as the prologue describes. I carry with me much gratitude for the queer women I have encountered in this research. Their self-representations shine a light on how we can overcome technological, social, economic, and political hurdles to reach out, connect, and rise up by sharing that which is personal to us.

NOTES

PROLOGUE
1. Depending on the time zone in which I was scrolling.
2. Facebook's API (application programming interface) once allowed for collecting network data pertaining to friends and friends-of-friends.
3. Although some of my childhood friends eventually came to identify as LGBTQ, none of them were out when we were growing up together. See chapter 1, note 1 for a discussion of my use of the term LGBTQ.

CHAPTER 1
1. I use *LGBTQ* when referring broadly to sexually and gender diverse people. I wrestle with this term, choosing it for its recognizability but noting how it joins the ranks of insufficient catch-alls that invisibilize those who fall outside or between the identities represented by these letters (Barker et al., 2009). The women I interviewed claimed a range of identities, including lesbian, gay, bisexual, transgender, and/or queer, to which I refer when writing about them individually. I also refer collectively to queer women, employing *queer* as a broad umbrella term that reflects its use by other scholars to indicate an identification at odds, or in tension, with heteronormativity (Gray, 2009; Warner, 1999).
2. For an exploration of how the family dinner table maintains and upkeeps normative roles and arrangements, see Sara Ahmed (2006).
3. Throughout the book, I differentiate between "public" as an adjective and as a noun. In terms of public as a quality of information, I examine how queer women adjust the publicness of their self-representations of sexual identity through identity modulation. Rarely do they share Tinder profiles, flirty selfies, or expressive videos in an unrestrained public manner. Instead, particular platforms and modes of targeting audiences establish boundaries constraining the degree to which these self-representations are public. When exchanging self-representations and related content, queer women are often participants in a public, as a thing: a gathering of people organized by discourse (Warner, 2002). Publics convene around discourse, with their boundaries demarcated by those who are able to access, attend to, share, and participate in such discourse. As boyd (2014) notes that publics convened through social media are shaped by networked technologies, I am interested in what shape publics take in relation to queer women's negotiation of app-specific affordances.
4. This book treats the notion of privacy in terms of interpersonal interaction rather than broader concerns regarding data privacy in relation to social media. There are many excellent examinations of corporate platforms' collection and use of personal data; see, for example, Kennedy (2016).

5. See Carmi (2020) for a compelling critique of the "overwhelming focus in the media and communication field . . . on vision, (in)visibility and seeing as ways to theorize and conceptualize power and ways of knowing, especially when it comes to new media" (p. 6). She proposes a shift to sound-related concepts, such as listening and rhythm, to examine power relations in the context of new media.

CHAPTER 2

1. "Netflix and chill" is an innuendo for visiting another person's house for hooking up, whether or not this includes watching television through the streaming service (Rickett, 2015).
2. Much of this line of thought was developed in conversation with Ben Light, who has written about delegation in relation to platforms like Ashley Madison (Light, 2016).
3. Such as those that take place on the Tinder subreddit at https://www.reddit.com/r/Tinder/.

CHAPTER 3

1. In conveying these interviews, I have chosen to represent participants' gender identities and pronouns as they were at the time of data collection. This allows for discussing the findings in their particular context at this specific point in participants' historical biographies. See the Appendix for further discussion of this decision and details about the range of interview participants.
2. See Alison Hearn and Sarah Banet-Weiser (2020) for an account of how the aesthetic category of glamour functions as a heuristic of platformized cultural production more broadly.
3. While the description of Instagram in this book is necessarily tailored for its relevance to identity modulation, see Leaver, Highfield, and Abidin (2020) for a thorough history and examination of the platform's affordances and user cultures.
4. Quotes and references to Vine's company materials are taken from my observational notes, as these materials are no longer available on the web and the app has been discontinued.
5. While "Do It for the Vine" was also the title of a hip-hop song, its widespread adoption as a catchphrase can largely be attributed to @Dom's video, which received 543,000 likes and 592,000 shares in just five months following its debut (Know Your Meme, 2016). Vine's adoption of the phrase without explicit links to @Dom replicates the common occurrence of corporations appropriating terms and phrases from Black culture without attributing their originators. Another well-known example of this appropriation involves Viner Peaches Monroee, whose phrase "on fleek" was used by multiple companies to sell products without compensation or attribution (St. Felix, 2015).
6. In 2019, hate groups co-opted the "OK emoji," and the Anti-Defamation League added it to a list of hate symbols (BBC News, 2019).
7. Neurodivergence can be understood as "the broad spectrum of neurocognitive functioning that significantly differs from what is considered 'normative'" (Logan, 2020).
8. For example, the teenage creators of the "Damn Daniel" viral Vine, in which one says to the other, "Damn Daniel! Back at it again with the white Vans," gained notoriety and a lifetime supply of Vans shoes from appearing on *The Ellen DeGeneres Show* (Regna, 2016). However, given subsequent controversies

regarding DeGeneres's friendships with former US presidents George W. Bush and Donald Trump as well as accusations that she perpetuated a toxic work environment (Hogan, 2021), being featured on her show or social media would no longer carry the same level of clout among LGBTQ audiences as it once did.

CHAPTER 4

1. While Tinder's features for individualized partner selection and one-on-one interaction preclude the formation of in-app publics, there are broader publics that gather in relation to shared practices and discourses pertaining to the app. These include publics of people who discuss their Tinder use, such as friends who help each other set up profiles, as well as publics of media commentators, bloggers, dating "experts" who give tips about the app, and others who produce discourse relating to it. The app has also sporadically introduced features that go beyond a one-on-one focus, such as "Tinder Social" that allowed groups of up to four users to swipe on each other but was discontinued in 2017, and an in-app game called "Swipe Night" that is available to all users within a specific location to spur discussion among them. However, neither of these has been an enduring interface feature.
2. Described in chapter 3.
3. As mentioned in the appendix, API research tools functioned in somewhat of a gray area regarding platform policies when this research was conducted in 2015. Instagram introduced a new review process for third-party apps in 2016, which Rieder (2016) engaged with in attempts to have the Instagram tool officially approved for research purposes. Unfortunately, it was declined without much explanation. Such decisions on the part of platforms, which have intensified following the Cambridge Analytica scandal, are understandable in light of calls to protect user data but leave researchers with no valid avenue for big picture social media analysis. Since researchers are bound to ethics protocols and the protection of individuals implicated in research, Rieder and others have called on platforms to develop avenues for scholars to be able to conduct research in the public interest independent of platform companies' influence (i.e., outside company-led and -controlled calls for research proposals). See, for example, the open letter composed by Axel Bruns (2018) and signed by a large number of academic researchers.
4. For a thorough understanding of Tumblr's affordances, user practices, and cultures, especially those giving rise to the development of overlapping NSFW and queer communities, see the collection edited by Allison McCracken, Alexander Cho, Louisa Stein, and Indira Neill Hoch (2020) and the book *Tumblr* by Katrin Tiidenberg, Crystal Abidin, and Natalie Ann Hendry (2021).

CONCLUSION

1. Despite the *New York Times*'s capitalization, girl in red prefers her name in lowercase.
2. Thanks to Kath Albury for drawing this connection.
3. This is an expansion on media scholar Jenny Sundén's (2003) original observation, later cited by boyd (2014), that individuals must write (or type) themselves into being to build an online presence, referring mainly to text-based online technologies.
4. One example of differential treatment of social media users, which is yet to be addressed through platforms' ad hoc policy making, includes the removal of

Instagram stories users posted on May 5, 2021, the National Day of Awareness for Missing and Murdered Indigenous Women and Girls in Canada and the United States (Boutsalis, 2021). While celebrity Dan Levy shared a post that remained on Instagram, many posts by Indigenous women and other users disappeared. Although a company representative asserted that the problem was due to a widespread issue and not related to this particular topic, Instagram's failure to protect groups who have experienced violence sees no end. Platforms like Instagram, and its parent company Facebook, fail to deploy effective policies to protect these users despite growing outcry about the frequent, unexplained removal of content created by marginalized groups.

5. The controversial US Fight Online Sex Trafficking Act (FOSTA) and Stop Enabling Sex Traffickers Act (SESTA) were signed into law in 2018, making internet intermediaries responsible for content posted pertaining to sex trafficking, often expanded to sex work-related content in general, as an exception to Section 230 of the Communications Decency Act (Romano, 2018).

6. Paasonen's talk, "Intimate Governance and the Value of Sex in Social Media," was hosted by the Department of Art History and Communication Studies at McGill University on January 23, 2020.

REFERENCES

Abidin, C. (2016). "Aren't these just young, rich women doing vain things online?": Influencer selfies as subversive frivolity. *Social Media + Society*, 2(2), 1–17. https://doi.org/10.1177/2056305116641342

Abidin, C. (2018). *Internet celebrity*. Emerald Publishing.

Abidin, C., & Cover, R. (2019). Gay, famous and working hard on YouTube: Influencers, queer microcelebrity publics and discursive activism. In P. Aggleton, R. Cover, D. Leahy, D. Marshall, & M. Rasumussen (Eds.), *Youth, sexuality and sexual citizenship* (pp. 217–231). Routledge.

Ahlm, J. (2016). Respectable promiscuity: Digital cruising in an era of queer liberalism. *Sexualities*, 20(3), 364–379. https://doi.org/10.1177/1363460716665783

Ahmed, S. (2006). *Queer phenomenology: Orientations, objects, others*. Duke University Press.

Albury, K. (2015). Selfies, sexts, and sneaky hats: Young people's understandings of gendered practices of self-representation. *International Journal of Communication*, 9, 1734–1745.

Albury, K. (2016). Politics of sexting revisited. In A. McCosker, S. Vivienne, & A. Johns (Eds.), *Negotiating digital citizenship: Control, contest and culture* (pp. 213–230). Rowman & Littlefield.

Albury, K. (2018). Heterosexual casual sex: From free love to Tinder. In C. Smith, F. Attwood, & B. McNair (Eds.), *The Routledge companion to media, sex and sexuality* (pp. 81–90). Routledge.

Albury, K., Burgess, J., Light, B., Race, K., & Wilken, R. (2017). Data cultures of mobile dating and hook-up apps: Emerging issues for critical social science research. *Big Data & Society*, 4(2), 1–11. https://doi.org/10.1177/2053951717720950

Alexander, J., & Losh, E. (2010). "A YouTube of one's own?": "Coming out" videos as rhetorical action. In C. Pullen & M. Cooper (Eds.), *LGBT identity and online new media* (pp. 37–50). Routledge.

Almeida, J., Johnson, R. M., Corliss, H. L., Molnar, B. E., & Azrael, D. (2009). Emotional distress among LGBT youth: The influence of perceived discrimination based on sexual orientation. *Journal of Youth and Adolescence*, 38(7), 1001–1014. https://doi.org/10.1007/s10964-009-9397-9

Alper, M. (2014). War on Instagram: Framing conflict photojournalism with mobile photography apps. *New Media & Society*, 16(8), 1233–1248. https://doi.org/10.1177/1461444813504265

Anderson, B. (1983). *Imagined communities*. Verso.

Anderson, M., Vogels, E. A., & Turner, E. (2020). *The virtues and downsides of online dating*. Pew Research Center. https://www.pewresearch.org/internet/2020/02/06/the-virtues-and-downsides-of-online-dating/

Anderson, T. L. (2005). Relationships among Internet attitudes, Internet use, romantic beliefs, and perceptions of online romantic relationships. *Cyberpsychology & Behaviour*, *8*(6), 521–531.

Ashley, B. (2020, July 13). Why Instagram influencers are unionising. *Vogue Business*. https://www.voguebusiness.com/companies/why-instagram-influencers-are-unionising

Baculinao, E. (2020, January 7). *Why is China raising the prospect of same-sex marriage?* NBC News. https://www.nbcnews.com/feature/nbc-out/why-china-raising-prospect-same-sex-marriage-n1109471

Banet-Weiser, S. (2012). *Authentic(TM): The politics of ambivalence in a brand culture*. New York University Press.

Banet-Weiser, S. (2018). *Empowered: Popular feminism and popular misogyny*. Duke University Press.

Barker, M., Richards, C., & Bowes-Catton, H. (2009). "All the world is queer save thee and ME . . .": Defining queer and bi at a critical sexology seminar. *Journal of Bisexuality*, *9*(3–4), 363–379.

Barnhurst, K. G. (2007). Visibility as paradox: Representation and simultaneous contrast. In K. G. Barnhurst (Ed.), *Media queered: Visibility and its discontents* (pp. 1–22). Peter Lang.

Baym, N. K. (2015). *Personal connections in the digital age* (2nd edition). Polity Press.

Baym, N. K. (2018). *Playing to the crowd: Musicians, audiences, and the intimate work of connection*. New York University Press.

BBC News. (2019, September 27). *OK hand sign added to list of hate symbols*. https://www.bbc.com/news/newsbeat-49837898

Beauman, F. (2011). *Shapely ankle preferr'd: A history of the lonely hearts ad*. Chatto & Windus.

Bengali, S. (2021, January 15). Facebook banned Trump but has failed to react quickly to other leaders who incited violence. *Los Angeles Times*. https://www.latimes.com/world-nation/story/2021-01-15/facebook-social-media-bans-trump-capitol-riot

Benkler, Y. (2006). *The wealth of networks: How social production transforms markets and freedom*. Yale University Press.

Bennett, S. (2013). *Visualizing Vine—Key stats, facts & figures for Twitter's video app*. Adweek. https://www.adweek.com/performance-marketing/vine-stats/

Berger, R. (2013). Now I see it, now I don't: Researcher's position and reflexivity in qualitative research. *Qualitative Research*, *15*(2), 219–234.

Berlant, L. (2008). *The female complaint: The unfinished business of sentimentality in American culture*. Duke University Press.

Berlant, L., & Warner, M. (1998). Sex in public. *Critical Inquiry*, *24*(2), 547–566.

Berry, D. M. (2011). The computational turn: Thinking about the digital humanities. *Culture Machine*, *12*, 1–22. https://doi.org/10.1007/s12599-014-0342-4

Biddle, S., Ribeiro, P. V., & Dias, T. (2020, March 16). *Invisible censorship*. The Intercept. https://theintercept.com/2020/03/16/tiktok-app-moderators-users-discrimination/

Bishop, S. (2018). Anxiety, panic and self-optimization: Inequalities and the YouTube algorithm. *Convergence, 24*(1), 69–84. https://doi.org/10.1177/1354856517736978

Bivens, R., & Haimson, O. L. (2016). Baking gender into social media design: How platforms shape categories for users and advertisers. *Social Media + Society, 2*(4), 1–12. https://doi.org/10.1177/2056305116672486

Blackwell, C., Birnholtz, J., & Abbott, C. (2015). Seeing and being seen: Co-situation and impression formation using Grindr, a location-aware gay dating app. *New Media & Society, 17*(7), 1117–1136. https://doi.org/10.1177/1461444814521595

Boboltz, S. (2015). *A brief history of "f**kboy," the Internet's favorite new man-bashing slur.* Huffington Post. http://www.huffingtonpost.com.au/entry/f--kboy-definition-take-that-haters_n_7471142

Bogle, K. A. (2008). *Hooking up: Sex, dating, and relationships on campus.* New York University Press.

Botella, E. (2019, December 4). *TikTok admits it suppressed videos by disabled, queer, and fat creators.* Slate. https://slate.com/technology/2019/12/tiktok-disabled-users-videos-suppressed.html

Boutsalis, K. (2021, May 7). *Instagram Stories about violence against Indigenous women are disappearing.* Vice. https://www.vice.com/en/article/jg8843/instagram-stories-about-mmiwg-violence-against-indigenous-women-are-disappearing

boyd, d. (2011). Social network sites as networked publics: Affordances, dynamics, and implications. In Z. Papacharissi (Ed.), *A networked self: Identity, community, and culture on social network sites* (pp. 39–58). Routledge.

boyd, d. (2014). *It's complicated: The social lives of networked teens.* Yale University Press.

Brickman, B. J. (2016). This charming butch: The male pop idol, girl fans, and lesbian (in)visibility. *Journal of Popular Music Studies, 28*(4), 443–459. http://doi.wiley.com/10.1111/jpms.12193

Brock, A. (2012). From the blackhand side: Twitter as a cultural conversation. *Journal of Broadcasting & Electronic Media, 56*(4), 529–549. https://doi.org/10.1080/08838151.2012.732147

Brock, A. (2020). *Distributed Blackness: African American cybercultures.* New York University Press.

Brock, R. (2014, January 2). *Tinder thumb.* Urban Dictionary. Retrieved August 1, 2019, from https://www.urbandictionary.com/define.php?term=Tinder Thumb

Brubaker, J. R., Ananny, M., & Crawford, K. (2016). Departing glances: A sociotechnical account of "leaving" Grindr. *New Media & Society, 18*(3), 373–390. https://doi.org/10.1177/1461444814542311

Bruns, A. (2008). *Blogs, Wikipedia, Second Life, and beyond: From production to produsage.* Peter Lang.

Bruns, A. (2018, April 25). *Facebook shuts the gate after the horse has bolted, and hurts real research in the process.* Internet Policy Review. https://policyreview.info/articles/news/facebook-shuts-gate-after-horse-has-bolted-and-hurts-real-research-process/786

Bruns, A., & Burgess, J. (2015). Twitter hashtags from ad hoc to calculated publics. In N. Rambukkana (Ed.), *Hashtag publics: The power and politics of discursive networks* (pp. 13–28). Peter Lang.

Bucher, T. (2012). Want to be on the top? Algorithmic power and the threat of invisibility on Facebook. *New Media & Society, 14*(7), 1164–1180. https://doi.org/10.1177/1461444812440159

Bucher, T. (2018). *If . . . then: Algorithmic power and politics*. Oxford University Press.

Bucher, T., & Helmond, A. (2017). The affordances of social media platforms. In J. Burgess, T. Poell, & A. Marwick (Eds.), *The Sage handbook of social media* (pp. 233–253). Sage.

Burgess, J. (2006). Hearing ordinary voices: Cultural studies, vernacular creativity and digital storytelling. *Continuum: Journal of Media & Cultural Studies, 20*(2), 201–214. https://doi.org/10.1080/10304310600641737

Butler, J. (1990). *Gender trouble: Feminism and the subversion of identity*. Routledge.

Byron, P. (2019). "How could you write your name below that?": The queer life and death of Tumblr. *Porn Studies, 6*(3), 336–349. https://doi.org/10.1080/23268743.2019.1613925

Calhoun, K. (2019). Vine racial comedy as anti-hegemonic humor: Linguistic performance and generic innovation. *Journal of Linguistic Anthropology, 29*(1), 27–49. https://doi.org/10.1111/jola.12206

Campbell, J. E. (2004). *Getting it on online: Cyberspace, gay male sexuality, and embodied identity*. Routledge.

Caplan, R., & Gillespie, T. (2020). Tiered governance and demonetization: The shifting terms of labor and compensation in the platform economy. *Social Media + Society, 6*(2), 1–13. https://doi.org/10.1177/2056305120936636

Carmi, E. (2020). *Media distortions: Understanding the power behind spam, noise, and other deviant media*. Peter Lang.

Carrasco, M., & Kerne, A. (2018). Queer visibility: Supporting LGBT+ selective visibility on social media. *Proceedings of the 2018 CHI Conference on Human Factors in Computing Systems*, 1–12. https://doi.org/10.1145/3173574.3173824

Carter, D. (2016). Hustle and brand: The sociotechnical shaping of influence. *Social Media + Society, 2*(3), 1–12. https://doi.org/10.1177/2056305116666305

Cassidy, E. (2018). *Gay men, identity and social media: A culture of participatory reluctance*. Routledge.

Castells, M. (2009). *Communication power*. Oxford University Press.

Castle, T. (1993). *The apparitional lesbian*. Columbia University Press.

Cavalcante, A. (2016). "I did it all online": Transgender identity and the management of everyday life. *Critical Studies in Media Communication, 33*(1), 109–122. https://doi.org/10.1080/15295036.2015.1129065

CBC Radio. (2019, January 11). *Why the Tumblr ban on "adult content" is bad for LGBTQ youth*. https://www.cbc.ca/radio/spark/spark-421-1.4973383/why-the-tumblr-ban-on-adult-content-is-bad-for-lgbtq-youth-1.4973385

Chandler, L., & Livingston, D. (2016). Reframing the authentic: Photography, mobile technologies and the visual language of digital imperfection. In M. Heitkemper-Yates & K. Kaczmarczyk (Eds.), *Learning to see: The meanings, modes and methods of visual literacy* (pp. 227–245). Brill.

Chaplin, T. (2014). Lesbians online: Queer identity and community formation on the French Minitel. *Journal of the History of Sexuality, 23*(3), 451–472. https://doi.org/10.7560/JHS23305

Chappell, B. (2018, April 16). *Weibo bans gay content—And quickly reverses itself after an outcry*. NPR. https://www.npr.org/sections/thetwo-way/2018/04/16/602902197/weibo-bans-gay-content-and-quickly-reverses-itself-after-an-outcry

Chen, S. (2018, June 1). *China's complicated LGBT movement*. The Diplomat. https://thediplomat.com/2018/06/chinas-complicated-lgbt-movement/

Chen, X., Kaye, D. B. V., & Zeng, J. (2020). #PositiveEnergy Douyin: Constructing "playful patriotism" in a Chinese short-video application. *Chinese Journal of Communication*, 1–21. https://doi.org/10.1080/17544750.2020.1761848

Cheney-Lippold, J. (2017). *We are data: Algorithms and the making of our digital selves*. New York University Press.

Cho, A. (2015). Queer reverb: Tumblr, affect, time. In K. Hillis, S. Paasonen, & M. Petit (Eds.), *Networked affect* (pp. 43–58). MIT Press.

Cho, A. (2017). Default publicness: Queer youth of color, social media, and being outed by the machine. *New Media & Society*, *20*(9), 1–18. https://doi.org/10.1177/1461444817744784

Clegg, N. (2021, June 4). *In response to Oversight Board, Trump suspended for two years; will only be reinstated if conditions permit*. Facebook Newsroom. https://about.fb.com/news/2021/06/facebook-response-to-oversight-board-recommendations-trump/

Cohen, C. J. (2005). Punks, bulldaggers, and welfare queens: The radical potential of queer politics. In E. P. Johnson & M. G. Henderson (Eds.), *Black queer studies: A critical anthology* (pp. 21–51). Duke University Press.

Colledge, L., Hickson, F., Reid, D., & Weatherburn, P. (2015). Poorer mental health in UK bisexual women than lesbians: Evidence from the UK 2007 Stonewall Women's Health Survey. *Journal of Public Health*, *37*(3), 427–437. https://doi.org/10.1093/pubmed/fdu105

CollegeHumor. (2014, January 29). *Tinderella: A modern fairy tale* [Video]. YouTube. https://youtu.be/bLoRPielarA

Combahee River Collective. (1986). *The Combahee River Collective statement: Black Feminist organizing in the seventies and eighties*. Kitchen Table.

Constine, J. (2016). *Founder's comment on Vine shutting down? "Don't sell your company!"* TechCrunch. https://techcrunch.com/2016/10/27/do-it-for-the-why/

Correll, S. (1995). The ethnography of an electronic bar: The Lesbian Cafe. *Journal of Contemporary Ethnography*, *24*(3), 270–298. https://doi.org/10.1177/089124195024003002

Couldry, N. (2010). *Why voice matters: Culture and politics after neoliberalism*. Sage.

Cover, R. (2019). Competing contestations of the norm: Emerging sexualities and digital identities. *Continuum: Journal of Media & Cultural Studies*, *33*(5), 602–613. https://doi.org/10.1080/10304312.2019.1641583

Craw, V. (2014, March 17). *The real story behind hugely successful dating app Tinder*. News.com.au. http://www.news.com.au/finance/business/the-real-story-behind-hugely-successful-dating-app-tinder/story-fn5lic6c-1226856885645

Crawford, K., & Gillespie, T. (2016). What is a flag for? Social media reporting tools and the vocabulary of complaint. *New Media & Society*, *18*(3), 410–428. https://doi.org/10.1177/1461444814543163

Crenshaw, K. (1991). Mapping the margins: Intersectionality, identity politics, and violence against women of color. *Stanford Law Review*, *43*(6), 1241–1299. https://doi.org/10.2307/1229039

Cunningham, S., & Craig, D. (2017). Being "really real" on YouTube: Authenticity, community and brand culture in social media entertainment. *Media International Australia*, *164*(1), 71–81. https://doi.org/10.1177/1329878X17709098

Cunningham, S., & Craig, D. (2019). *Social media entertainment: The new intersection of Hollywood and Silicon Valley*. New York University Press.

Curtis, C. (2019, December 5). *Twitter to introduce stricter content NSFW guidelines—Worrying adult content creators.* The Next Web. https://thenextweb.com/tech/2019/12/05/twitter-to-follow-facebook-and-instagram-with-new-anti-nsfw-guidelines/

Daily Mail. (2015, April 22). Kristen Stewart gets touchy-feely with her live-in gal pal Alicia Cargile as they celebrate star's 25th birthday at Coachella. https://www.dailymail.co.uk/tvshowbiz/article-3046645/Inseparable-Kristen-Stewart-enjoys-Coachella-live-gal-pal-Alicia-Cargile-three-days-25th-birthday.html#ixzz4YCfzWCSL

Daniels, J. (2009). Rethinking cyberfeminism(s): Race, gender, and embodiment. *WSQ: Women's Studies Quarterly*, 37(1 & 2), 101–124.

Daroya, E. (2018). "Not into chopsticks or curries": Erotic capital and the psychic life of racism on Grindr. In D. W. Riggs (Ed.), *The psychic life of racism in gay men's communities*. Lexington Books.

David, G., & Cambre, C. (2016). Screened intimacies: Tinder and the swipe logic. *Social Media + Society*, 2(2), 1–11. https://doi.org/10.1177/2056305116641976

Davies, H. C., & Eynon, R. (2018). Is digital upskilling the next generation our "pipeline to prosperity"? *New Media & Society*, 20(11), 3961–3979. https://doi.org/10.1177/1461444818783102

Davis, J. L., & Jurgenson, N. (2014). Context collapse: Theorizing context collusions and collisions. *Information, Communication & Society*, 17(4), 476–485. https://doi.org/10.1080/1369118X.2014.888458

de Lauretis, T. (1993). Sexual indifference and lesbian representation. In H. Abelove, M. Barale, & D. Haperin (Eds.), *The gay and lesbian studies reader* (pp. 141–158). Routledge.

de Souza e Silva, A. (2006). From cyber to hybrid: Mobile technologies as interfaces of hybrid spaces. *Space and Culture*, 9(3), 261–278. https://doi.org/10.1177/1206331206289022

Deleuze, G. (1992). Postscript on the societies of control. *October*, 59(Winter), 3–7.

DeSantis, A. D. (2007). *Inside Greek U.: Fraternities, sororities, and the pursuit of pleasure, power, and prestige.* University Press of Kentucky.

DeVito, M. A., Walker, A. M., & Birnholtz, J. (2018). "Too gay for Facebook": Presenting LGBTQ+ identity throughout the personal social media ecosystem. *Proceedings of the ACM on Human-Computer Interaction*, 2(CSCW), 1–23. https://doi.org/10.1145/3274313

Diamond, L. M. (2005). "I'm straight but I kissed a girl": The trouble with American media representations of female-female sexuality. *Feminism & Psychology*, 15(1), 104–110. https://doi.org/10.1177/0959353505049712

Dias, A. (2019, March 6). *"I thought Australia was safe": At least four LGBTI people assaulted on Mardi Gras weekend.* ABC News. https://www.abc.net.au/triplej/programs/hack/mardi-gras-assault-four-lgbt-men-sydney/10872014

Dobson, A. S. (2015). *Postfeminist digital cultures: Femininity, social media, and self-representation.* Palgrave Macmillan.

Dockray, H. (2019, June 27). *The best Pride Month memes of 2019.* Mashable. https://mashable.com/article/best-pride-month-memes-2019/

D'Onofrio, J. (2018). *A better, more positive Tumblr.* Tumblr Staff. https://staff.tumblr.com/post/180758987165/a-better-more-positive-tumblr

Duffy, B. E. (2016). The romance of work: Gender and aspirational labour in the digital culture industries. *International Journal of Cultural Studies*, 19(4), 441–457. https://doi.org/10.1177/1367877915572186

Duffy, B. E. (2017). *(Not) getting paid to do what you love: Gender, social media, and aspirational work*. Yale University Press.

Duffy, B. E., & Wissinger, E. (2017). Mythologies of creative work in the social media age: Fun, free, and "just being me." *International Journal of Communication, 11*, 4652–4671. http://ijoc.org/index.php/ijoc/article/view/7322

Duggan, L. (2002). The new homonormativity: The sexual politics of neoliberalism. In R. Castronovo & D. D. Nelson (Eds.), *Materializing democracy: Toward a revitalized culture politics* (pp. 175–194). Duke University Press.

Duguay, S. (2016a). "He has a way gayer Facebook than I do": Investigating sexual identity disclosure and context collapse on a social networking site. *New Media & Society, 18*(6), 891–907. https://doi.org/10.1177/1461444814549930

Duguay, S. (2016b). Lesbian, gay, bisexual, trans, and queer visibility through selfies: Comparing platform mediators across Ruby Rose's Instagram and Vine presence. *Social Media + Society, 2*(2), 1–12. https://doi.org/10.1177/2056305116641975

Duguay, S. (2017). Dressing up Tinderella: Interrogating authenticity claims on the mobile dating app Tinder. *Information, Communication & Society, 20*(3), 351–367. https://doi.org/10.1080/1369118X.2016.1168471

Duguay, S. (2018). Swiped: A focal gesture and contested app visions. In J. W. Morris & S. Murray (Eds.), *Appified: Culture in the age of apps* (pp. 127–135). University of Michigan Press.

Duguay, S. (2019). "Running the numbers": Modes of microcelebrity labor in queer women's self-representation on Instagram and Vine. *Social Media + Society, 5*(4), 1–11. https://doi.org/10.1177/2056305119894002

Duguay, S. (2020). You can't use this app for that: Exploring off-label use through an investigation of Tinder. *The Information Society, 36*(1), 30–42. https://doi.org/10.1080/01972243.2019.1685036

Duguay, S., Burgess, J., & Suzor, N. (2018). Queer women's experiences of patchwork platform governance on Tinder, Instagram, and Vine. *Convergence: The International Journal of Research into New Media Technologies, 26*(2), 237–252. https://doi.org/10.1177/1354856518781530

Duportail, J., Kayser-Bril, N., Schacht, K., & Richard, E. (2020, June 15). *Undress or fail: Instagram's algorithm strong-arms users into showing skin*. AlgorithmWatch. https://algorithmwatch.org/en/story/instagram-algorithm-nudity/

Dyer, H. T. (2020). *Designing the social: Unpacking social media design and identity*. Springer.

Eppink, J. (2014). A brief history of the GIF (so far). *Journal of Visual Culture, 13*(3), 298–306. https://doi.org/10.1177/1470412914553365

Eynon, R., & Geniets, A. (2016). The digital skills paradox: How do digitally excluded youth develop skills to use the internet? *Learning, Media and Technology, 41*(3), 463–479. https://doi.org/10.1080/17439884.2014.1002845

Facebook. (2019, May 16). *Using surveys to make News Feed more personal*. Facebook Newsroom. Retrieved August 12, 2020, from https://newsroom.fb.com/news/2019/05/more-personalized-experiences/

Farvid, P., & Aisher, K. (2016). "It's just a lot more casual": Young heterosexual women's experience of using Tinder in New Zealand. *Ada: A Journal of Gender, New Media, and Technology, 10*. http://adanewmedia.org/2016/10/issue10-farvid-aisher/

Feiner, L. (2020, June 23). *Twitter flagged another Trump tweet for violating its policies*. CNBC. https://www.cnbc.com/2020/06/23/twitter-labeled-another-trump-tweet-for-violating-its-policies.html

Ferguson, M. (2016, June 30). *Why OITNB refuses to say the word "bisexual."* Pride. https://www.pride.com/oitnb/2016/6/30/why-oitnb-refuses-say-word-bisexual

Ferris, L., & Duguay, S. (2019). Tinder's lesbian digital imaginary: Investigating (im)permeable boundaries of sexual identity on a popular dating app. *New Media & Society, 22*(3), 489–506. https://doi.org/10.1177/1461444819864903

Fink, M., & Miller, Q. (2014). Trans media moments: Tumblr, 2011–2013. *Television & New Media, 15*(7), 611–626. https://doi.org/10.1177/1527476413505002

Florini, S. (2014). Tweets, Tweeps, and signifyin': Communication and cultural performance on "Black Twitter." *Television & New Media, 15*(3), 223–237. https://doi.org/10.1177/1527476413480247

Foucault, M. (1990). *The history of sexuality: Vol. 1. An introduction* (R. Hurley, Trans.). Vintage Books. (Original work published in 1978).

Fowler, G. (2020, July 13). Is it time to delete TikTok? A guide to the rumors and the real privacy risks. *The Washington Post.* https://www.washingtonpost.com/technology/2020/07/13/tiktok-privacy/

Franzke, A., Bechmann, A., Zimmer, M., & Ess, C. (2019). *Internet research: Ethical guidelines 3.0.* Association of Internet Researchers. https://aoir.org/reports/ethics3.pdf

Fraser, N. (1990). Rethinking the public sphere: A contribution to the critique of actually existing democracy. *Social Text, 25/26,* 56–80.

Frolic, A. N. (2001). Wear it with pride: The fashions of Toronto's pride parade and Canadian queer identities. In T. Goldie (Ed.), *In a queer country: Gay and lesbian studies in the Canadian context* (pp. 264–291). Arsenal Pulp Press.

Fuchs, C. (2010). Labor in informational capitalism and on the Internet. *The Information Society, 26*(3), 179–196. https://doi.org/10.1080/01972241003712215

Fuchs, C., & Dyer-Witheford, N. (2013). Karl Marx @ internet studies. *New Media & Society, 15*(5), 782–796. https://doi.org/10.1177/1461444812462854

Gehl, R. W. (2014). *Reverse engineering social media: Software, culture, and political economy in new media capitalism.* Temple University Press.

Gehl, R. W., Moyer-Horner, L., & Yeo, S. K. (2017). Training computers to see internet pornography: Gender and sexual discrimination in computer vision science. *Television and New Media, 18*(6), 529–547. https://doi.org/10.1177/1527476416680453

Gercio, H. (2015). *Looking for that "special" lady: Exploring hegemonic masculinity in online dating profiles of trans-attracted men.* Central European University.

Gerlitz, C., & Helmond, A. (2013). The like economy: Social buttons and the data-intensive web. *New Media & Society, 15*(8), 1348–1365. https://doi.org/10.1177/1461444812472322

Gerrard, Y., & Thornham, H. (2020). Content moderation: Social media's sexist assemblages. *New Media & Society, 22*(7), 1266–1286. https://doi.org/10.1177/1461444820912540

Ghaziani, A. (2014). *There goes the gayborhood?* Princeton University Press.

Gibbs, J. L., Ellison, N. B., & Lai, C.-H. (2011). First comes love, then comes Google: An investigation of uncertainty reduction strategies and self-disclosure in online dating. *Communication Research, 38*(1), 70–100. https://doi.org/10.1177/0093650210377091

Gibbs, M., Meese, J., Arnold, M., Nansen, B., & Carter, M. (2016). #Funeral and Instagram: Death, social media, and platform vernacular. *Information,*

Communication & Society, 18(3), 255–268. https://doi.org/10.1080/1369118X.2014.987152

Gibson, J. J. (1979). *The ecological approach to visual perception*. Psychology Press.

Gillespie, T. (2012). The relevance of algorithms. In T. Gillespie, P. J. Boczkowski, & K. A. Foot (Eds.), *Media technologies: Essays on communication, materiality, and society* (pp. 167–194). MIT Press.

Gillespie, T. (2013, July 26). *Tumblr, NSFW porn blogging, and the challenge of checkpoints*. Culture Digitally. http://culturedigitally.org/2013/07/tumblr-nsfw-porn-blogging-and-the-challenge-of-checkpoints/

Gillespie, T. (2015). Platforms intervene. *Social Media + Society*, 1(1), 1–2. https://doi.org/10.1177/2056305115580479

Gillespie, T. (2018). *Custodians of the internet: Platforms, content moderation, and the hidden decisions that shape social media*. Yale University Press.

Gillett, R. (2018). Intimate intrusions online: Studying the normalisation of abuse in dating apps. *Women's Studies International Forum*, 69, 212–219. https://doi.org/10.1016/j.wsif.2018.04.005

Gleason, B. (2018). Adolescents becoming feminist on Twitter: New literacies practices, commitments, and identity work. *International Literacy Association*, 62(3), 281–289. https://doi.org/10.1002/jaal.889

Goffman, E. (1959). *The presentation of self in everyday life*. Doubleday.

Goffman, E. (1963). *Stigma: Notes on the management of a spoiled identity*. Simon & Schuster.

Goffman, E. (1966). *Behavior in public places: Notes on the social organization of gatherings*. Simon & Schuster.

Goldblum, P., Testa, R. J., Pflum, S., Hendricks, M. L., Bradford, J., & Bongar, B. (2012). The relationship between gender-based victimization and suicide attempts in transgender people. *Professional Psychology: Research and Practice*, 43(5), 468–475. https://doi.org/10.1037/a0029605

Goldhaber, M. (1997). The attention economy and the net. *First Monday*, 2(4). https://doi.org/10.5210/fm.v2i4.519

Gonzales, G., Przedworski, J., & Henning-Smith, C. (2016). Comparison of health and health risk factors between lesbian, gay, and bisexual adults and heterosexual adults in the United States. *JAMA Internal Medicine*, 176(9), 1344–1351. https://doi.org/10.1001/jamainternmed.2016.3432

Gorwa, R., Binns, R., & Katzenbach, C. (2020). Algorithmic content moderation: Technical and political challenges in the automation of platform governance. *Big Data & Society*, 7(1), 1–15. https://doi.org/10.1177/2053951719897945

Gray, M. L. (2009). *Out in the country: Youth, media, and queer visibility in rural America*. New York University Press.

Gross, L. (2001). *Up from invisibility: Lesbians, gay men, and the media in America*. Columbia University Press.

Gudelunas, D. (2012). There's an app for that: The uses and gratifications of online social networks for gay men. *Sexuality & Culture*, 16(4), 347–365. https://doi.org/10.1007/s12119-012-9127-4

Haas, A. P., Eliason, M., Mays, V. M., Mathy, R. M., Cochran, S. D., D'Augelli, A. R., Silverman, M. M., Fisher, P. W., Hughes, T., Rosario, M., Russell, S. T., Malley, E., Reed, J., Litts, D. A., Haller, E., Sell, R. L., Remafedi, G., Bradford, J., Beautrais, A. L., . . . Clayton, P. J. (2010). Suicide and suicide risk in lesbian, gay, bisexual, and transgender populations: Review and recommendations.

Journal of Homosexuality, 58(1), 10–51. https://doi.org/10.1080/00918369.2011.534038

Haimson, O. L., Dame-Griff, A., Capello, E., & Richter, Z. (2019). Tumblr was a trans technology: The meaning, importance, history, and future of trans technologies. *Feminist Media Studies*, 1–17. https://doi.org/10.1080/14680777.2019.1678505

Halavais, A. (2014). Structure of Twitter: Social and technical. In K. Weller, A. Bruns, J. Burgess, M. Mahrt, & C. Puschmann (Eds.), *Twitter and society* (pp. 29–42). Peter Lang.

Hanckel, B., Vivienne, S., Byron, P., Robards, B., & Churchill, B. (2019). "That's not necessarily for them": LGBTIQ+ young people, social media platform affordances and identity curation. *Media, Culture & Society, 41*(8), 1261–1278. https://doi.org/10.1177/0163443719846612

Hargittai, E., & Hsieh, Y. P. (2013). Digital inequality. In W. H. Dutton (Ed.), *The Oxford handbook of internet studies* (pp. 129–150). Oxford University Press.

Harper, D. (2002). Talking about pictures: A case for photo elicitation. *Visual Studies, 17*(1), 13–26. https://doi.org/10.1080/14725860220137345

Harris, K. (2019, April 16). *New gay rights coin divides LGBT community and outrages social conservatives*. CBC News. https://www.cbc.ca/news/politics/mint-coin-loonie-homosexual-rights-1.5095317

Haythornthwaite, C. (2005). Social networks and Internet connectivity effects. *Information, Communication & Society, 8*(2), 125–147. https://doi.org/10.1080/13691180500146185

Hearn, A. (2010). Structuring feeling: Web 2.0, online ranking and rating, and the digital "reputation" economy. *Ephemera: Theory & Politics in Organization, 10*(3/4), 421–438.

Hearn, A., & Banet-Weiser, S. (2020). The beguiling: Glamour in/as platformed cultural production. *Social Media + Society, 6*(1), 1–11. https://doi.org/10.1177/2056305119898779

Herrera, A. P. (2017). Theorizing the lesbian hashtag: Identity, community, and the technological imperative to name the sexual self. *Journal of Lesbian Studies, 22*(3), 313–328. https://doi.org/10.1080/10894160.2018.1384263

Hesmondhalgh, D. (2010). User-generated content, free labour and the cultural industries. *Ephemera: Theory & Politics in Organization, 10*(3/4), 267–284.

Hess, A., & Flores, C. (2018). Simply more than swiping left: A critical analysis of toxic masculine performances on Tinder Nightmares. *New Media & Society, 20*(3), 1085–1102. https://doi.org/10.1177/1461444816681540

Highfield, T., & Duguay, S. (2015). "Like a monkey with a miniature cymbal": Cultural practices of repetition in visual social media. *AoIR Selected Papers of Internet Research, 5*. https://spir.aoir.org/ojs/index.php/spir/article/view/8446

Highfield, T., & Leaver, T. (2015). A methodology for mapping Instagram hashtags. *First Monday, 20*(1). https://doi.org/10.5210/fm.v20i1.5563

Hightower, J. L. (2015). Producing desirable bodies: Boundary work in a lesbian niche dating site. *Sexualities, 18*(1–2), 20–36. https://doi.org/10.1177/1363460714550900

Hjorth, L., & Lim, S. S. (2012). Mobile intimacy in an age of affective mobile media. *Feminist Media Studies, 12*(4), 477–484. https://doi.org/10.1080/14680777.2012.741860

Hogan, B. (2010). The presentation of self in the age of social media: Distinguishing performances and exhibitions online. *Bulletin of Science, Technology & Society*, *30*(6), 377–386. https://doi.org/10.1177/0270467610385893

Hogan, H. (2021, May 12). *Ellen DeGeneres is ending her talk show amid endless backlash (but reportedly not because of backlash)*. Autostraddle. https://www.autostraddle.com/ellen-degeneres-is-ending-her-talkshow/

Hopper. (2019). *Instagram rich list 2019*. Retrieved June 18, 2020, from https://www.hopperhq.com/blog/instagram-rich-list/

Hunt, S. (2018). Foreword. In Q. Eades & S. Vivienne (Eds.), *Going postal: More than "yes" or "no."* Brow Books.

Instagram. (2015). *Community guidelines*. Retrieved November 6, 2015, from https://help.instagram.com/477434105621119/

Instagram. (2020). *Community guidelines*. Retrieved August 16, 2020, from https://help.instagram.com/477434105621119

Jackson, S., & Gilbertson, T. (2009). 'Hot lesbians': Young people's talk about representations of lesbianism. *Sexualities*, *12*(2), 199–224. https://doi.org/10.1177/1363460708100919

Jarrett, K. (2015). *Feminism, labour and digital media: The digital housewife*. Routledge.

Jenefsky, C., & Miller, D. H. (1998). Phallic intrusion: Girl-girl sex in *Penthouse*. *Women's Studies International Forum*, *21*(4), 375–385. https://doi.org/10.1016/S0277-5395(98)00042-9

Jenkins, H. (2006). *Convergence culture: Where old and new media collide*. New York University Press.

Jenkins, H., Ford, S., & Green, J. (2013). *Spreadable media: Creating value and meaning in a networked culture*. New York University Press.

Jin, D. Y. (2015). *Digital platforms, imperialism and political culture*. Routledge.

Josephs, B. (2016, October 28). Here's every time a Vine made us love a song. *Spin*. https://www.spin.com/2016/10/musical-moments-vine/

Kanai, A. (2016). Sociality and classification: Reading gender, race, and class in a humorous meme. *Social Media + Society*, *2*(4), 1–12. https://doi.org/10.1177/2056305116672884

Kanai, A. (2019). *Gender and relatability in digital culture: Managing affect, intimacy and value*. Palgrave Macmillan.

Kaplan, K. A. (2003, November 19). Facemash creator survives Ad Board. *Harvard Crimson*. http://www.thecrimson.com/article/2003/11/19/facemash-creator-survives-ad-board-the/

Kavada, A. (2015). Social media as conversation: A manifesto. *Social Media + Society*, *1*(1), 1–2. https://doi.org/10.1177/2056305115580793

Keating, S. (2019, December 5). *"The L Word: Generation Q" is trying to atone for the original's sins*. BuzzFeed News. https://www.buzzfeednews.com/article/shannonkeating/l-word-generation-q-showtime-tales-of-the-city-lesbian

Kennedy, H. (2016). *Post, mine, repeat: Social media data mining becomes ordinary*. Palgrave Macmillan.

Kerr, D. L., Santurri, L., & Peters, P. (2013). A comparison of lesbian, bisexual, and heterosexual college undergraduate women on selected mental health issues. *Journal of American College Health*, *61*(4), 185–194. https://doi.org/10.1080/07448481.2013.787619

Know Your Meme. (2016). *Do it for the Vine*. Retrieved January 10, 2017, from http://knowyourmeme.com/memes/do-it-for-the-vine

Kohn, A. (2015). Instagram as a naturalized propaganda tool: The Israel Defense Forces Web site and the phenomenon of shared values. *Convergence: The International Journal of Research into New Media Technologies, 23*(2), 197–213. https://doi.org/10.1177/1354856515592505

Krishna, R. (2018, December 4). *Tumblr launched an algorithm to flag porn and so far it's just caused chaos.* BuzzFeed News. https://www.buzzfeednews.com/article/krishrach/tumblr-porn-algorithm-ban

Lange, P. G. (2007). Publicly private and privately public: Social networking on YouTube. *Journal of Computer-Mediated Communication, 13*(1), 361–380. https://doi.org/10.1111/j.1083-6101.2007.00400.x

Lange, P. G. (2009). Videos of affinity. In P. Snickas & P. Vonderau (Eds.), *The YouTube reader* (pp. 70–88). National Library of Sweden.

Langford, S. (2019, January 7). *Junk explained: What the hell is TikTok, and is it the new Vine?* Junkee. https://junkee.com/tiktok-app-vine-challenge/188567

Lapowsky, I. (n.d.). How Tinder is winning the mobile dating wars. *Inc.* https://www.inc.com/issie-lapowsky/how-tinder-is-winning-the-mobile-dating-wars.html

Latour, B. (1992). Where are the missing masses? The sociology of a few mundane artifacts. In W. E. Bijker & J. Law (Eds.), *Shaping technology/building society: Studies in sociotechnical change* (pp. 227–254). MIT Press.

Latour, B. (2005). *Reassembling the social: An introduction to actor-network-theory.* Oxford University Press.

Leaver, T. (2015). Born digital? Presence, privacy, and intimate surveillance. In J. Hartley & W. Qu (Eds.), *Re-orientation: Translingual, transcultural, transmedia: Studies in narrative, language, identity, and knowledge* (pp. 149–160). Fudan University Press.

Leaver, T., Highfield, T., & Abidin, C. (2020). *Instagram.* Polity.

Lee, C. (2015, August 13). Trap kings: How the hip-hop sub-genre dominated the decade. *The Guardian.* https://www.theguardian.com/music/2015/aug/13/trap-kings-how-hip-hop-sub-genre-dominated-decade

Leonard, W., Lyons, A., & Bariola, E. (2015). *A closer look at private lives 2: Addressing the mental health and well-being of lesbian, gay, bisexual and transgender (LGBT) Australians.* La Trobe University.

Leong, L. (2016). Mobile identities: Managing self and stigma in iPhone app use. *Observatorio, 10*(1), 1–25.

Liao, S. (2019, March 14). *After the porn ban, Tumblr users have ditched the platform as promised.* The Verge. https://www.theverge.com/2019/3/14/18266013/tumblr-porn-ban-lost-users-down-traffic

Licoppe, C., Riviere, C. A., & Morel, J. (2016). Grindr casual hook-ups as interactional achievements. *New Media & Society, 18*(11), 2540–2558. https://doi.org/10.1177/1461444815589702

Light, A. (2011). HCI as heterodoxy: Technologies of identity and the queering of interaction with computers. *Interacting with Computers, 23*(5), 430–438. https://doi.org/10.1016/j.intcom.2011.02.002

Light, B. (2016). The rise of speculative devices: Hooking up with the bots of Ashley Madison. *First Monday, 21*(6). https://doi.org/10.5210/fm.v21i6.6426

Light, B., Burgess, J., & Duguay, S. (2018). The walkthrough method: An approach to the study of apps. *New Media & Society, 20*(3), 881–900. https://doi.org/10.1177/1461444816675438

Lim, S. S., Vadrevu, S., Chan, Y. H., & Basnyat, I. (2012). Facework on Facebook: The online publicness of juvenile delinquents and youths-at-risk. *Journal of*

Broadcasting & Electronic Media, 56(3), 346–361. https://doi.org/10.1080/
08838151.2012.705198

Lingel, J., & Golub, A. (2015). In face on Facebook: Brooklyn's drag community
and sociotechnical practices of online communication. *Journal of Computer-
Mediated Communication, 20*(5), 536–553. https://doi.org/10.1111/jcc4.12125

Lippmann, W. (1922). *Public opinion.* Harcourt, Brace and Company.

Litt, E. (2012). Knock, knock: Who's there? The imagined audience. *Journal of
Broadcasting & Electronic Media, 56*(3), 330–345. https://doi.org/10.1080/
08838151.2012.705195

Little, M., & Hollister, S. (2017, August 15). *Reddit, Facebook ban neo-Nazi
groups after Charlottesville attack.* CNET. https://www.cnet.com/news/
reddit-facebook-bans-neo-nazi-groups-charlottesville-attack/

Liu, J. (2021). The carceral feminism of SESTA-FOSTA: Reproducing spaces of
exclusion from IRL to URL. In R. Ramos & S. Mowlabocus (Eds.), *Queer sites in
global contexts: Technologies, spaces, and otherness* (pp. 117–132). Routledge.

Livia, A. (2002). Public and clandestine: Gay men's pseudonyms on the
French Minitel. *Sexualities, 5*(2), 201–217. https://doi.org/10.1177/
1363460702005002004

Livingstone, S. (2008). Taking risky opportunities in youthful content
creation: Teenagers' use of social networking sites for intimacy, privacy and
self-expression. *New Media & Society, 10*(3), 393–411. https://doi.org/10.1177/
1461444808089415

Logan, J. (2020). Queer and neurodivergent identity production within the
social media panopticon. *The Macksey Journal, 1*(177), 1–24. https://www.
mackseyjournal.org/publications/vol1/iss1/177

Lorenz, T. (2016, October 29). *"We knew Vine was dead"—Vine's biggest stars tried
to save the company, but they were ignored.* Business Insider. http://www.
businessinsider.com/vines-biggest-stars-tried-saving-company-2016-
10?IR=T

Lovelock, M. (2017). "Is every YouTuber going to make a coming out video
eventually?": YouTube celebrity video bloggers and lesbian and gay
identity. *Celebrity Studies, 8*(1), 87–103. https://doi.org/10.1080/
19392397.2016.1214608

Luka, M. E., & Millette, M. (2018). (Re)framing big data: Activating situated
knowledges and a feminist ethics of care in social media research. *Social Media
+ Society, 4*(2), 1–10. https://doi.org/10.1177/2056305118768297

Lyric. (2004). *Lipstick lesbian.* Urban Dictionary. Retrieved August 13, 2019, from
https://www.urbandictionary.com/define.php?term=lipstick lesbian

Lytle, M. C., De Luca, S. M., & Blosnich, J. R. (2014). The influence of intersecting
identities on self-harm, suicidal behaviors, and depression among lesbian, gay,
and bisexual individuals. *Suicide and Life-Threatening Behavior, 44*(4), 384–391.
https://doi.org/10.1111/sltb.12083

MacKee, F. (2016). Social media in gay London: Tinder as an alternative to hook-up
apps. *Social Media + Society, 2*(3). https://doi.org/10.1177/2056305116662186

Mackenzie, D., & Wajcman, J. (Eds.). (1999). *The social shaping of technology* (2nd
edition). Open University Press.

Madden, S. (2015, February 10). The best fan Vines of Fetty Wap's "Trap Queen." *XXL.*
https://www.xxlmag.com/the-best-trap-queen-vines/

Mangan, D., & Breuninger, K. (2020, May 26). *Twitter fact-checks Trump, slaps warning
labels on his tweets about mail-in ballots.* CNBC. https://www.cnbc.com/2020/05/

26/twitter-fact-checks-trump-slaps-warning-labels-on-his-tweets-about-mail-in-ballots.html

Marinova, P. (2016, August 9). How Tinder used Greek life for more than just hookups. *Fortune.* https://fortune.com/2016/08/09/entrepreneurs-greek-life-tinder/

Marone, V. (2017). Looping out loud: A multimodal analysis of humour on Vine. *The European Journal of Humour Research, 4*(4), 50–66. https://doi.org/10.7592/ejhr2016.4.4.marone

Marwick, A. E. (2015). Instafame: Luxury selfies in the attention economy. *Public Culture, 27*(1), 137–160. https://doi.org/10.1215/08992363-2798379

Marwick, A. E. (2016). You may know me from YouTube: (Micro-)celebrity in social media. In P. D. Marshall & S. Redmond (Eds.), *A companion to celebrity* (pp. 333–350). Wiley.

Marwick, A. E., & boyd, d. (2011). I tweet honestly, I tweet passionately: Twitter users, context collapse, and the imagined audience. *New Media & Society, 13*(1), 114–133. https://doi.org/10.1177/1461444810365313

Marwick, A. E., & boyd, d. (2014). Networked privacy: How teenagers negotiate context in social media. *New Media & Society, 16*(7), 1051–1067. https://doi.org/10.1177/1461444814543995

Marwick, A. E., & Lewis, R. (2017, May 15). *Media manipulation and disinformation online.* Data & Society. https://datasociety.net/output/media-manipulation-and-disinfo-online/

Massanari, A. (2015). #Gamergate and the Fappening: How Reddit's algorithm, governance, and culture support toxic technocultures. *New Media & Society, 19*(3), 329–346. https://doi.org/10.1177/1461444815608807

Matamoros-Fernández, A. (2017). Platformed racism: The mediation and circulation of an Australian race-based controversy on Twitter, Facebook and YouTube. *Information, Communication & Society, 20*(6), 930–946. https://doi.org/10.1080/1369118X.2017.1293130

McBean, S. (2016). The "gal pal epidemic." *Celebrity Studies, 7*(2), 282–284. https://doi.org/10.1080/19392397.2016.1165005

McCracken, A., Cho, A., Stein, L., Hoch, I. N. (Eds.). (2020). *A Tumblr book: Platforms and cultures.* University of Michigan Press.

McGlotten, S. (2013). *Virtual intimacies: Media, affect and queer sociality.* SUNY Press.

McKee, A. (2003). *Textual analysis: A beginner's guide.* Sage.

McNaron, T. A. H. (2007). Post-lesbian? Not yet. *Journal of Lesbian Studies, 11*(1–2), 145–151. https://doi.org/10.1300/J155v11n01_10

McVeigh-Schultz, J., & Baym, N. K. (2015). Thinking of you: Vernacular affordance in the context of the microsocial relationship app, Couple. *Social Media + Society, 1*(2), 1–13. https://doi.org/10.1177/2056305115604649

Meese, J., Gibbs, M., & Kohn, T. (2015). Selfies at funerals: Mourning and presencing on social media platforms. *International Journal of Communication, 9,* 1818–1831.

Mercuri, M. (2018, August 2). Musical.ly merges with new video app TikTok, creating single global platform. *Billboard.* https://www.billboard.com/articles/business/8468281/musically-merges-tiktok-bytedance.

Merriam-Webster. (n.d.). *What is a 'thirst trap'? A tall drink of water.* Words We're Watching. https://www.merriam-webster.com/words-at-play/what-is-a-thirst-trap

Meyrowitz, J. (1985). *No sense of place: The impact of electronic media on social behavior.* Oxford University Press.

Michelson, N. (2017, March 17). *We need to talk about WTF is up with Kristen Stewart's sexuality.* Huffington Post. https://www.huffingtonpost.ca/entry/kristen-stewart-bisexual_n_58cabd70e4b00705db4cf1b5

Miller, V. (2008). New media, networking and phatic culture. *Convergence: The International Journal of Research into New Media Technologies, 14*(4), 387–400. https://doi.org/10.1177/1354856508094659

Miltner, K. M. (2018). Internet memes. In J. Burgess, A. Marwick, & T. Poell (Eds.), *The Sage handbook of social media* (pp. 412–428). Sage.

Miltner, K. M. (2020). "One part politics, one part technology, one part history": Racial representation in the Unicode 7.0 emoji set. *New Media & Society,* 1–20. https://doi.org/10.1177/1461444819899623

Mohammed-baksh, S., & Callison, C. (2015). Hegemonic masculinity in hip-hop music? Difference in brand mention in rap music based on the rapper's gender. *Journal of Promotion Management, 21*(3), 351–370. https://doi.org/10.1080/10496491.2015.1039177

Morris, M., & Anderson, E. (2015). "Charlie is so cool like": Authenticity, popularity and inclusive masculinity on YouTube. *Sociology, 49*(6), 1200–1217. https://doi.org/10.1177/0038038514562852

Morse, J., & Richards, L. (2002). *Read me first for a user's guide to qualitative research.* Sage.

Mossberger, K., Tolbert, C. J., & McNeal, R. S. (2008). *Digital citizenship: The internet, society, and participation.* MIT Press.

Mowlabocus, S. (2010). *Gaydar culture: Gay men, technology and embodiment in the digital age.* Ashgate.

Nagy, P., & Neff, G. (2015). Imagined affordance: Reconstructing a keyword for communication theory. *Social Media + Society, 1*(2), 1–9. https://doi.org/10.1177/2056305115603385

Nakamura, L. (2002). *Cybertypes: Race, ethnicity, and identity on the Internet.* Routledge.

Nash, C. J. (2013). The age of the "post-mo"? Toronto's gay Village and a new generation. *Geoforum, 49,* 243–252. https://doi.org/10.1016/j.geoforum.2012.11.023

Newett, L., Churchill, B., & Robards, B. (2017). Forming connections in the digital era: Tinder, a new tool in young Australian intimate life. *Journal of Sociology, 54*(3), 346–361. https://doi.org/10.1177/1440783317728584

Newton, C. (2020, June 29). *Reddit bans r/The_Donald and r/ChapoTrapHouse as part of a major expansion of its rules.* The Verge. https://www.theverge.com/2020/6/29/21304947/reddit-ban-subreddits-the-donald-chapo-trap-house-new-content-policy-rules

Ng, E. (2013). A "post-gay" era? Media gaystreaming, homonormativity, and the politics of LGBT integration. *Communication, Culture & Critique, 6*(2), 258–283. https://doi.org/10.1111/cccr.12013

Nieborg, D. B., & Poell, T. (2018). The platformization of cultural production: Theorizing the contingent cultural commodity. *New Media & Society, 20*(11), 4275–4292. https://doi.org/10.1177/1461444818769694

Nissenbaum, H. (2009). *Privacy in context: Technology, policy, and the integrity of social life.* Stanford University Press.

Noble, S. U. (2018). *Algorithms of oppression: How search engines reinforce racism*. New York University Press.

Norcie, G., De Cristofaro, E., & Bellotti, V. (2013). Bootstrapping trust in online dating: Social verification of online dating profiles. *Lecture Notes in Computer Science*, 7862, 149–163.

Norman, D. A. (1988). *The psychology of everyday things*. Basic Books.

Nunez, C. (2016, June 16). Map shows where being LGBT can be punishable by law. *National Geographic*. http://news.nationalgeographic.com/2016/06/lgbt-laws-gay-rights-world-map/

O'Brien, S. A. (2017, March 11). *Tinder's Sean Rad: App has made 250,000 transgender matches*. CNN. https://money.cnn.com/2017/03/10/technology/sxsw-tinder-glaad/index.html

Odell, J. (2019). *How to do nothing: Resisting the attention economy*. Melville House.

OkCupid. (2019). Privacy controls. Retrieved August 1, 2019, from https://help.okcupid.com/article/143-privacy-controls

Olszanowski, M. (2014). Feminist self-imaging and Instagram: Tactics of circumventing sensorship. *Visual Communication Quarterly*, 21(2), 83–95. https://doi.org/10.1080/15551393.2014.928154

Olszanowski, M. (2015). The 1x1 common: The role of Instagram's hashtag in the development and maintenance of feminist exchange. In N. Rambukkana (Ed.), *Hashtag publics: The power and politics of discursive networks* (pp. 229–242). Peter Lang.

O'Riordan, K. (2005). From Usenet to Gaydar: A comment on queer online community. *SIGGROUP Bulletin*, 25(2), 28–32. https://doi.org/10.1145/1067721.1067727

Orne, J. (2011). "You will always have to 'out' yourself": Reconsidering coming out through strategic outness. *Sexualities*, 14(6), 681–703. https://doi.org/10.1177/1363460711420462

Orne, J. (2017). *Boystown: Sex and community in Chicago*. University of Chicago Press.

Paasonen, S., Jarrett, K., & Light, B. (2019). *#NSFW: Sex, humor, and risk in social media*. MIT Press.

Papacharissi, Z. (2009). The virtual geographies of social networks: A comparative analysis of Facebook, LinkedIn and ASmallWorld. *New Media & Society*, 11(1–2), 199–220. https://doi.org/10.1177/1461444808099577

Papacharissi, Z., & Gibson, P. L. (2011). Fifteen minutes of privacy: Privacy, sociality and publicity on social network sites. In S. Trepte & L. Reinecke (Eds.), *Privacy online* (pp. 75–89). Springer-Verlag Berlin Heidelberg. https://doi.org/10.1007/978-3-642-21521-6

Parkin, S. (2018, September 8). The YouTube stars heading for burnout: "The most fun job imaginable became deeply bleak." *The Guardian*. https://www.theguardian.com/technology/2018/sep/08/youtube-stars-burnout-fun-bleak-stressed

Pelias, R. J. (2011). Writing into position: Strategies for composition and evaluation. In N. K. Denzin & Y. S. Lincoln (Eds.), *The Sage handbook of qualitative research* (pp. 659–668). Sage.

Perrin, A., & Monica, A. (2019, April 10). *Share of U.S. adults using social media, including Facebook, is mostly unchanged since 2018*. Pew Research Center. https://www.pewresearch.org/fact-tank/2019/04/10/share-of-u-s-adults-using-social-media-including-facebook-is-mostly-unchanged-since-2018/

Peterson, T. (2013, January 24). *Twitter resurrects video sharing apps with Vine launch*. AdWeek. http://www.adweek.com/news/technology/twitter-resurrects-video-sharing-apps-vine-launch-146752

Pham, S. (2020, May 5). *TikTok is winning over millennials and Instagram stars as its popularity explodes*. CNN. https://www.cnn.com/2020/05/05/tech/tiktok-bytedance-coronavirus-intl-hnk/index.html

Phillips, W. (2015). *This is why we can't have nice things: Mapping the relationship between online trolling and mainstream culture*. MIT Press.

Plummer, K. (1996). Symbolic interactionism and the forms of homosexuality. In S. Seidman (Ed.), *Queer theory/sociology* (pp. 64–82). Blackwell.

Plummer, K. (2003). *Intimate citizenship: Private decisions and public dialogues*. McGill-Queen's University Press.

Pond, T., & Farvid, P. (2017). "I do like girls, I promise": Young bisexual women's experiences of using Tinder. *Psychology of Sexualities Review, 8*(2), 6–24.

Quiroz, P. A. (2013). From finding the perfect love online to satellite dating and "loving-the-one-you're near": A look at Grindr, Skout, Plenty of Fish, Meet Moi, Zoosk and Assisted Serendipity. *Humanity & Society, 37*(2), 181–185. https://doi.org/10.1177/0160597613481727

Race, K. (2015). Speculative pragmatism and intimate arrangements: Online hook-up devices in gay life. *Culture, Health & Sexuality, 17*(4), 37–41.

Rainie, L., & Wellman, B. (2012). *Networked: The new social operating system*. MIT Press.

Raun, T. (2018). Capitalizing intimacy: New subcultural forms of micro-celebrity strategies and affective labour on YouTube. *Convergence, 24*(1), 99–113. https://doi.org/10.1177/1354856517736983

Raynes-Goldie, K. (2010). Aliases, creeping, and wall cleaning: Understanding privacy in the age of Facebook. *First Monday, 15*(1–4). https://doi.org/10.5210/fm.v15i1.2775

Regna, M. (2016, February 24). *"Damn, Daniel" was on "Ellen" and it was amazing*. BuzzFeed. https://www.buzzfeed.com/michelleregna/damn-daniel-was-on-ellen#.gswR11LRr

Reilly, A., & Saethre, E. J. (2013). The hankie code revisited: From function to fashion. *Critical Studies in Men's Fashion, 1*(1), 69–78.

Renninger, B. J. (2015). "Where I can be myself . . . where I can speak my mind": Networked counterpublics in a polymedia environment. *New Media & Society, 17*(9), 1513–1529. https://doi.org/10.1177/1461444814530095

Richards, L. (2009). *Handling qualitative data: A practical guide* (2nd ed.). Sage.

Richardson, D. (1998). Sexuality and citizenship. *Sociology, 32*(1), 83–100.

Richardson, D. (2005). Desiring sameness? The rise of a neoliberal politics of normalisation. *Antipode, 37*(3), 515–535. https://doi.org/10.1111/j.0066-4812.2005.00509.x

Richardson, D. (2018). *Sexuality and citizenship*. Polity.

Rickett, O. (2015, September 29). How "Netflix and chill" became code for casual sex. *The Guardian*. https://www.theguardian.com/media/shortcuts/2015/sep/29/how-netflix-and-chill-became-code-for-casual-sex

Rieder, B. (2016, May 27). *Closing APIs and the public scrutiny of very large online platforms*. The Politics of Systems. http://thepoliticsofsystems.net/2016/05/closing-apis-and-the-public-scrutiny-of-very-large-online-platforms/

Riotta, C. (2019, July 17). Tinder still banning transgender people despite pledge of inclusivity. *Independent*. https://www.independent.co.uk/news/world/

americas/tinder-ban-trans-account-block-report-lawsuit-pride-gender-identity-a9007721.html

Robards, B., Churchill, B., Vivienne, S., Hanckel, B., & Byron, P. (2018). Twenty years of "cyberqueer": The enduring significance of the Internet for young LGBTIQ+ people. In P. Aggleton, R. Cover, D. Leahy, D. Marshall, & M. L. Rasmussen (Eds.), *Youth, sexuality and sexual citizenship* (pp. 151–167). Routledge.

Robards, B., & Lincoln, S. (2016). Making it "Facebook official": Reflecting on romantic relationships through sustained Facebook use. *Social Media + Society*, 2(4), 1–10. https://doi.org/10.1177/2056305116672890

Robards, B., & Lincoln, S. (2017). Uncovering longitudinal life narratives: Scrolling back on Facebook. *Qualitative Research*, 17(6), 715–730. https://doi.org/10.1177/1468794117700707

Roberts, S. (2019). *Behind the screen: Content moderation in the shadows of social media.* Yale University Press.

Rogers, R. (2013). *Digital methods.* MIT Press.

Romano, A. (2018, July 2). *A new law intended to curb sex trafficking threatens the future of the internet as we know it.* Vox. https://www.vox.com/culture/2018/4/13/17172762/fosta-sesta-backpage-230-internet-freedom

Rose, G. (2012). *Visual methodologies: An introduction to the interpretation of visual methods* (3rd ed.). Sage.

Roth, Y. (2015). "No overly suggestive photos of any kind": Content management and the policing of self in gay digital communities. *Communication, Culture & Critique*, 8(3), 414–432. https://doi.org/10.1111/cccr.12096

Sales, N. J. (2015, August 31). Tinder and the dawn of the "dating apocalypse." *Vanity Fair*. http://www.vanityfair.com/culture/2015/08/tinder-hook-up-culture-end-of-dating

Schiermer, B. (2014). Late-modern hipsters: New tendencies in popular culture. *Acta Sociologica*, 57(2), 167–181. https://doi.org/10.1177/0001699313498263

Sedgwick, E. K. (1990). *Epistemology of the closet.* University of California Press.

Seiter, E. (2017). Stereotype. In L. Ouellette & J. Gray (Eds.), *Keywords for media studies* (pp. 184–185). New York University Press.

Senft, T. M. (2008). *Camgirls: Celebrity and community in the age of social networks.* Peter Lang.

Senft, T. M. (2013). Microcelebrity and the branded self. In J. Harley, J. Burgess, & A. Bruns (Eds.), *A companion to new media dynamics* (pp. 346–354). Blackwell.

Senft, T. M., & Baym, N. K. (2015). What does the selfie say? Investigating a global phenomenon. *International Journal of Communication*, 9, 1588–1606.

Sergi, V., & Bonneau, C. (2016). Making mundane work visible on social media: A CCO investigation of working out loud on Twitter. *Communication Research and Practice*, 2(3), 378–406. https://doi.org/10.1080/22041451.2016.1217384

Shaw, F. (2016). "Bitch I said hi": The Bye Felipe campaign and discursive activism in mobile dating apps. *Social Media + Society*, 2(4). https://doi.org/10.1177/2056305116672889

Shifman, L. (2014). *Memes in digital culture.* MIT Press.

Shontell, A. (2014, July 11). *Tinder, a $500 million dating app, used this pitch deck when it was just a tiny startup.* Business Insider. https://www.businessinsider.com/tinders-first-startup-pitch-deck-2014-7

Sinfield, A. (1998). *Gay and after.* Serpent's Tail.

Sismondo, S. (2010). *An introduction to science and technology studies* (2nd edition). Wiley-Blackwell.

Slone, I. (2020, March 10). Escape into cottagecore, calming ethos for our febrile moment. *The New York Times*. https://www.nytimes.com/2020/03/10/style/cottagecore.html

Smith, K. M., & Tyler, I. (2017). Lesbian brides: Post-queer popular culture. *Feminist Media Studies*, 1–17. https://doi.org/10.1080/14680777.2017.1282883

Southerton, C., Marshall, D., Aggleton, P., Rasmussen, M. L., & Cover, R. (2021). Restricted modes: Social media, content classification and LGBTQ sexual citizenship. *New Media & Society*, 23(5), 920-938. https://doi.org/10.1177/1461444820904362

Spez. (2020). *Update to our content policy*. Reddit. Retrieved July 23, 2020, from https://www.reddit.com/r/announcements/comments/hi3oht/update_to_our_content_policy/

Spišak, S., Pirjatanniemi, E., Paalanen, T., Paasonen, S., & Vihlman, M. (2021). Social networking sites' gag order: Commercial content moderation's adverse implications for fundamental sexual rights and wellbeing. *Social Media + Society*, 7(2), 1-9. https://doi.org/10.1177/20563051211024962

St. Felix, D. (2015, December 3). Black teens are breaking the internet and seeing none of the profits. *The Fader*. https://www.thefader.com/2015/12/03/on-fleek-peaches-monroee-meechie-viral-vines

Stampler, L. (2014, February 6). Inside Tinder: Meet the guys who turned dating into an addiction. *Time*. http://time.com/4837/tinder-meet-the-guys-who-turned-dating-into-an-addiction/

Stark, L., & Crawford, K. (2015). The conservatism of emoji: Work, affect, and communication. *Social Media + Society*, 1(2), 1–11. https://doi.org/10.1177/2056305115604853

Sterne, J., & Rodgers, T. (2011). The poetics of signal processing. *Differences*, 22(2–3), 31–53. https://doi.org/10.1215/10407391-1428834

Stuart, F. (2020). *Ballad of the bullet: Gangs, drill music, and the power of online infamy*. Princeton University Press.

Sundén, J. (2003). *Material virtualities: Approaching online textual embodiment*. Peter Lang.

Suzor, N. (2019). *Lawless: The secret rules that govern our digital lives*. Cambridge University Press.

Szulc, L., & Dhoest, A. (2013). The internet and sexual identity formation: Comparing Internet use before and after coming out. *The European Journal of Communication Research*, 38(4), 347–365.

Tait Communications. (2019). Modulation and radio building blocks. Retrieved July 12, 2019, from https://www.taitradioacademy.com/topic/how-does-modulation-work-1-1/

Tang, D. T. S. (2017). All I get is an emoji: Dating on lesbian mobile phone app Butterfly. *Media, Culture & Society*, 39(6), 816–832. https://doi.org/10.1177/0163443717693680

Terranova, T. (2000). Free labor: Producing culture for the digital economy. *Social Text*, 18(2), 33–58.

Thumim, N. (2012). *Self-representation and digital culture*. Palgrave Macmillan.

Tiidenberg, K. (2018). *Selfies: Why we love (and hate) them*. Emerald Publishing.

Tiidenberg, K., & Gomez Cruz, E. (2015). Selfies, image and the re-making of the body. *Body & Society*, 21(4), 77–102. https://doi.org/10.1177/1357034X15592465

Tiidenberg, K., Hendry, N. A., & Abidin, C. (2021). *Tumblr*. Polity.

Tiidenberg, K., & van der Nagel, E. (2020). *Sex and social media*. Emerald Publishing.

Tinder. (2019, March 15). *Powering Tinder—The method behind our matching*. Tinder Blog. Retrieved August 12, 2019, from https://blog.gotinder.com/powering-tinder-r-the-method-behind-our-matching/

Twitter Inc. (2021). *Permanent suspension of @realDonaldTrump*. Retrieved June 10, 2021, from https://blog.twitter.com/en_us/topics/company/2020/suspension.html

Unicode Inc. (2019). The Unicode Consortium. Retrieved July 10, 2019, from https://www.unicode.org/

Valdiserri, R. O., Holtgrave, D. R., Poteat, T. C., & Beyrer, C. (2019). Unraveling health disparities among sexual and gender minorities: A commentary on the persistent impact of stigma. *Journal of Homosexuality*, *66*(5), 571–589. https://doi.org/10.1080/00918369.2017.1422944

van Dijck, J. (2013). *The culture of connectivity: A critical history of social media*. Oxford University Press.

van Dijck, J., & Poell, T. (2013). Understanding social media logic. *Media and Communication*, *1*(1), 2. https://doi.org/10.17645/mac.v1i1.70

van Dijck, J., Poell, T., & de Waal, M. (2018). *The platform society*. Oxford University Press.

Veix, J. (2014). *I joined Tinder as a dog*. Death and Taxes. Retrieved June 1, 2014, from https://www.buzzfeed.com/richardhjames/man-joins-tinder-as-a-dog-gets-sent-some-pretty-bizarre-mess

Vine, L. (2018, April 5). *I'm addicted to dating apps—But I don't want a date*. BBC. https://www.bbc.co.uk/bbcthree/article/a0abe5ca-ad4b-4c08-8a10-a616480711ff

Vitak, J. (2012). The impact of context collapse and privacy on social network site disclosures. *Journal of Broadcasting & Electronic Media*, *56*(4), 451–470. https://doi.org/10.1080/08838151.2012.732140

Vivienne, S. (2016a). *Digital identity and everyday activism*. Palgrave Macmillan.

Vivienne, S. (2016b). Intimate citizenship 3.0. In A. McCosker, S. Vivienne, & A. Johns (Eds.), *Negotiating digital citizenship: Control, contest and culture* (pp. 147–166). Rowman & Littlefield.

Vivienne, S., McCosker, A., & Johns, A. (2016). Digital citizenship as fluid interface: Between control, contest and culture. In A. McCosker, S. Vivienne, & A. Johns (Eds.), *Negotiating digital citizenship: Control, contest and culture* (pp. 1–18). Rowman & Littlefield.

Wakeford, N. (1996). Sexualized bodies in cyberspace. In C. Warren, M. Deegan, & A. Gibson (Eds.), *Beyond the book: Theory, culture, and the politics of cyberspace* (pp. 93–104). University of London.

Walcott, R. (2017, June 28). *Black Lives Matter, police and Pride: Toronto activists spark a movement*. The Conversation. https://theconversation.com/black-lives-matter-police-and-pride-toronto-activists-spark-a-movement-79089

Ward, J. (2016). Swiping, matching, chatting: Self-presentation and self-disclosure on mobile dating apps. *Human IT*, *13*(2), 81–95.

Wargo, J. M. (2015). "Every selfie tells a story . . .": LGBTQ youth lifestreams and new media narratives as connective identity texts. *New Media & Society*, *19*(4), 560–578. https://doi.org/10.1177/1461444815612447

Warner, M. (1999). *The trouble with normal: Sex, politics, and the ethics of queer life*. Harvard University Press.

Warner, M. (2002). *Publics and counterpublics*. Zone Books.

Watkins, S. C. (2018). Introduction: The digital edge. In S. C. Watkins, A. Lombana-Bermudez, A. Cho, V. Shaw, J. Vickery, & L. Weinzimmer (Eds.), *The digital edge: How Black and Latino youth navigate digital equality* (pp. 1–18). New York University Press.

Watson, L. B., Morgan, S. K., & Craney, R. (2018). Bisexual women's discrimination and mental health outcomes: The roles of resilience and collective action. *Psychology of Sexual Orientation and Gender Diversity, 5*(2), 182–193. https://doi.org/10.1037/sgd0000272

West, S. M. (2017). Raging against the machine: Network gatekeeping and collective action on social media platforms. *Media and Communication, 5*(3), 28–36. https://doi.org/10.17645/mac.v5i3.989

Williams, R. (1977). *Marxism and literature.* Oxford University Press.

Wilson, L. (2020, June 29). For lesbians, TikTok is "the next Tinder." *The New York Times.* https://www.nytimes.com/2020/06/29/style/lesbian-tiktok-dating.html

Witt, A., Suzor, N., & Huggins, A. (2019). The rule of law on Instagram: An evaluation of the moderation of images depicting women's bodies. *University of New South Wales Law Journal, 42*(2), 557–596.

Worthen, M. G. F. (2016). Hetero-cis-normativity and the gendering of transphobia. *International Journal of Transgenderism, 17*(1), 31–57. https://doi.org/10.1080/15532739.2016.1149538

Xiao, S., Metaxa, D., Park, J. S., Karahalios, K., & Salehi, N. (2020). Random, messy, funny, raw: Finstas as intimate reconfigurations of social media. *CHI '20: Proceedings of the 2020 CHI Conference on Human Factors in Computing Systems,* 1–13. https://doi.org/10.1145/3313831.3376424

Zappavigna, M. (2016). Social media photography: Construing subjectivity in Instagram images. *Visual Communication, 15*(3), 271–292. https://doi.org/10.1177/1470357216643220

Zhao, S., Grasmuck, S., & Martin, J. (2008). Identity construction on Facebook: Digital empowerment in anchored relationships. *Computers in Human Behavior, 24*(5), 1816–1836. https://doi.org/10.1016/j.chb.2008.02.012

Zhao, X., Salehi, N., Naranjit, S., Alwaalan, S., Voida, S., & Cosley, D. (2013). The many faces of Facebook: Experiencing social media as performance, exhibition, and personal archive. *CHI'13: Proceedings of the SIGCHI Conference on Human Factors in Computing Systems,* 1–10. https://doi.org/10.1145/2470654.2470656

Zimmer, M. (2010). "But the data is already public": On the ethics of research in Facebook. *Ethics and Information Technology, 12*(4), 313–325. https://doi.org/10.1007/s10676-010-9227-5

INDEX

Instagram (*cont.*)
 publics on, 84–89
 self-branding on, 63–72, 114
InterActiveCorp (IAC), 37
Intercept, 107
Internet Relay Chat, 92
intersectionality, 3–4, 29, 93
intimacy. *See* mobile intimacy; naked
 intimacy
intimate affective labor, 30, 59, 64–66
intimate citizenship, 122–123, 125
intimate publics (Berlant concept), 83,
 85–86, 88

Jarrett, Kylie, 113–114, 120
Jaxx (interview subject), 69–72, 74,
 77–78, 93–94, 98–99, 115
Jin, Dal Yong, 19
Julia (interview subject), 41–42, 45–46, 50
Julie (interview subject), 69, 73–74,
 87–88, 96
Jurgenson, Nathan, 17

Kamala (interview subject), 68–69,
 74, 87
Kanai, Akane, 65, 110
Kavada, Anastasia, 24
Kelzz (interview subject), 66, 69, 71, 76,
 86
Kik, 96, 100
Krieger, Mike, 60
Kroll, Colin, 61

labor
 aspirational, 64, 71–72
 developmental aesthetic, 30, 59, 64,
 67–70
 intimate affective, 30, 59, 64–66
 relational, 59, 64, 72
Lange, Patricia, 89
Latinx people, 69, 111
Latour, Bruno, 52–53
Laura (interview subject), 43–44, 49–50
#lesbehonest, 56, 79, 89
#lesbian, 67, 87, 97, 116
Lesbian Cafe, 81
lesbian digital imaginary, 30, 47–49, 54,
 83, 110
lesbians. *See* queer women
#lesbiansofinstagram, 84

Lesbian TikTok, 105–108, 110
#LGBTCrew, 67, 89
LGBTQ people. *See* asexual people;
 bisexual people; gay men; gender
 nonconforming people; genderqueer
 people; pansexual people; queer
 women; transgender people
Light, Ann, 109, 124
Light, Ben, 26, 120, 134n2
like economy, 58. *See also* attention
 economy
Lim, Sun Sun, 16
LinkedIn, 57
lipstick lesbian, 47–48
listservs, 80–81, 104
Litt, Eden, 11–12
Livingston, Debra, 60
Lovelock, Michael, 78
lupus, 68–69
L Word: Generation Q, The, 85

manifest dismantling, 124–125
Marwick, Alice, 19, 61
Marxism, 77
Massanari, Adrienne, 98
Mastodon, 103
Mechanical Turk, 36
media multiplexity, 51–52
memes, 1–2, 21, 43, 62, 66, 111
methodology (of book), 25–29, 127–132,
 134n1
Meyrowitz, Joshua, 11–12, 53
microcelebrity, 57, 64–66, 71–72, 78,
 113–115. *See also* influencers
millennials, 43, 111
Minitel, 15
misinformation, 117–118
Mïta (interview subject), 67, 75, 86–87
mobile intimacy, 16, 53
modulation (Cheney-Lippold concept),
 5–6
modulation (sound). *See* sound
 modulation
#moonday, 63
Mozilla, 22
MSN Messenger, 52
Muff Diva Index (MDI), 80
Musical.ly, 105
My Little Pony, 63
MySpace, 11, 84

salience (*cont.*)
    dynamics of, 19–25, 108, 113, 119,
        122–123, 125
    and self-branding, 59, 64, 67, 72–73, 76
    on Tinder, 30, 35–36, 44–52, 54, 57
Sam and Alyssa (YouTubers), 85
same-sex marriage, 27–28, 106
Sappho listserv, 80–82, 104
Saturday Night Live, 46
Seiter, Ellen, 19
self-branding, 30, 57–64, 68, 72, 75, 78–
    79, 86, 113–114
self-representation
    definition of, 3–5
    digital, 25–26, 29, 53, 114, 119,
        125–126
    sexual, 120, 122
Senft, Theresa, 57
sexual citizenship, 121–122, 124
sexual sociability, 92, 98, 101
sex work, 120, 136n5
Shuler, Diamonique, 62–63, 90, 134n5
signal processing, 6, 13, 25
signifyin' (Florini concept), 81, 90
Silva, Adriana de Souza e, 37
Singapore, 69
Snapchat, 51, 96
social media. *See individual platforms*
social steganography, 19
sound modulation, 6, 56, 134n5. *See also*
    signal processing
Spotify, 39
Stanford University, 60
Stark, Luke, 21
Sterne, Jonathan, 6
Stewart, Kristen, 46, 49, 106
stigma (Goffman concept), 7–9, 11
strategic outness (Orne concept), 10
Stuart, Forrest, 71
subaltern counterpublics, 82. *See also*
    counterpublics
Suzor, Nicolas, 43, 97, 101, 115–116, 123
Sydney, Australia, 28
Systrom, Kevin, 60

techno-cultural constructs, 13
television. *See individual shows*
Terranova, Tiziana, 68, 77
Thailand, 68, 87
Thea (interview subject), 68, 75

#TheStrugglesofALesbian, 89
thirst trapping, 31, 91–92, 98, 121
ThunderGoddess (interview subject), 42,
    44, 50
Tiidenberg, Katrin, 120
TikTok, 26, 105–108, 110–111, 125–126
Tinder
    deception on, 40–44
    Facebook and, 18, 30, 32–35, 38–39,
        49–54, 111
    gender identification on, 48–49, 111
    heterosexuality of, 35–36, 40, 44
    personal identifiability on, 34–38, 49,
        51, 53–54, 109
    prepopulating identities, 36–39
    publics on, 83, 135n1
    reach on, 35–36, 49–51, 53–54
    salience on, 30, 35–36, 44–52, 54, 57
    See also lesbian digital imaginary
Tinderella: A Modern Fairy Tale (2014), 35
@tindernightmares, 43
toxic technocultures, 98–99, 119
transgender people
    discrimination against, 28
    on Facebook, 15–16
    fetishization of, 100
    inclusion in book, 3–4
    on Instagram, 70, 87
    media representations of, 113
    on Tinder, 48–49, 53, 111
    on Tumblr, 102
    vloggers, 65, 78
transphobia, 48–49, 53
"Trap Queen" (Fetty Wap song), 91
Trump, Donald, 117–118, 135n8
#ttsquad, 91
Tumblr, 68, 93–94, 102–104
Twilight (2008), 46
Twitter, 11, 61, 75, 77, 81–82, 92–93,
    104, 118

Unicode, 21, 45
unions, 115
United States, 18, 66, 91–92, 94, 117–118,
    120, 130, 136n4
Usenet, 81

van der Nagel, Emily, 120
van Dijck, José, 13, 18
Vanity Fair, 43